HARDCORE Neuroscience

HARDCORE Pharmacology

HARDCORE Neuroscience

HARDCORE Microbiology and Immunology

HARDCORE Pathology

HARDCORE Neuroscience

Kevin C. Wang, MD, PhD
Internal Medicine Resident
Brigham and Women's Hospital
Boston, Massachusetts
Dermatology Resident
University of California, San Francisco
San Francisco, California

Rita A. Mukhtar, BA
Class of 2006
University of California, San Francisco
School of Medicine
San Francisco, California

Series Editors:
Rodrigo E. Saenz, MD
Internal Medicine Resident
Louisiana State University Medical
Center
New Orleans, Louisiana

Benjamin W. Sears, MD
Orthopaedic Surgery Resident
Loyola University Medical Center
Chicago, Illinois

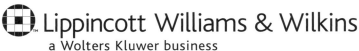
. Lippincott Williams & Wilkins
a Wolters Kluwer business
Philadelphia · Baltimore · New York · London
Buenos Aires · Hong Kong · Sydney · Tokyo

Acquisitions Editor: Nancy Duffy
Development Editor: Kathleen Scogna
Production Editor: Sirkka E.H. Bertling
Interior Designer: Janice Bielawa
Cover Designer: Shawn Girsberger
Compositor: Graphicraft Ltd. in Hong Kong
Printer: Walsworth Publishing Co.

Printed in the United States of America

Library of Congress Cataloging-in-Publication Data

Wang, Kevin C.
    Hardcore neuroscience / authors, Kevin C. Wang, Rita A. Mukhtar.
        p. ; cm. — (Hardcore series)
    ISBN-13: 978-1-4051-0471-5 (pbk. : alk. paper)
    ISBN-10: 1-4051-0471-6 (pbk. : alk. paper)   1. Neurosciences—Outlines, syllabi, etc.
  2. Nervous system—Diseases—Outlines, syllabi, etc.
        [DNLM: 1. Nervous System Physiology—Examination Questions.   2. Nervous
  System Physiology—Outlines.   3. Nervous System—anatomy & histology—Examination
  Questions.   4. Nervous System—anatomy & histology—Outlines.   5. Nervous System
  Diseases—Examination Questions.   6. Nervous System Diseases—Outlines. WL 18.2
  W246h 2006]   I. Mukhtar, Rita A.   II. Title.   III. Series.

    RC343.6.W36 2006
    612.8′076--dc22

                                                                         2005017380

To our families, friends, and loved ones,
and
our mentors and colleagues at UCSF

About the Authors

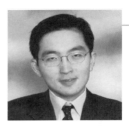

Kevin C. Wang

Kevin was born and raised in Taipei, Taiwan and grew up in the San Francisco Bay Area before attending Stanford University, where he graduated in 1997 with Bachelor of Science and Master of Science degrees in Biological Sciences. After a year character-building in Cambridge, UK as a Fulbright scholar, he began medical school at the University of California San Francisco (UCSF) School of Medicine, but withdrew in 2000 to begin graduate studies of mammalian axonal regeneration at Harvard Medical School. In his spare time as a graduate student Kevin participated in several editions of the review text *First Aid for the USMLE Step One*. Kevin obtained his Doctor of Philosophy degree in Neurobiology in 2003, returned to UCSF to complete the clinical portion of his medical training, and graduated with his Medical Doctorate degree in May 2005. After a subsequent sabbatical year as an intern at Brigham and Women's Hospital in Boston, he will return to UCSF to start his dermatology residency.

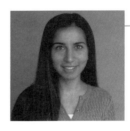

Rita A. Mukhtar

Rita grew up in San Jose, California and attended the University of California at Berkeley, where she graduated with a degree in Molecular and Cell Biology, and a minor in Music in 2000. She then moved across the Bay to begin her medical studies at UCSF in 2001. Currently, she is pursuing a year-long Doris Duke Clinical Research Fellowship, studying the effects of lipoproteins on the hepatocyte inflammatory response. She will graduate with her Medical Doctorate in May 2006.

A Note to the Reader

HARDCORE *Neuroscience* was developed with a similar intention as the **HARDCORE** *Pharmacology* book—to provide medical students preparing for USMLE Step 1 with an ultra high-yield neuroscience review **that was pared down to just the most heavily tested, "hardcore" facts**. To date, neuroscience remains one of the more difficult topics for which to prepare due to the overwhelming amount of information and the complexities of its clinical application, often requiring considerable effort on the part of the student to identify and then master the key concepts. We were struck by the lack of easily readable neuroscience texts available to students—most review books had *too much* information, and we were unable to find one good source that provided us with a comprehensive, easy-to-understand review of neuroscience and the necessary neuroanatomy.

Our neuroscience backgrounds and recent Step 1 experiences came together to develop this ultra high-yield neuroscience review book **that brings you the information that is actually tested on the board exam**.

GETTING HARDCORE

With so many areas to cover in writing a neuroscience review, we spent a great deal of time deciding how to balance the necessary fundamentals with the commonly tested clinical outcomes. We pored through a wide range of sources, from detailed textbooks to short review books, to identify information we agreed would be pertinent to Step 1. The result is a book that begins with fundamentals, covering neurophysiology and anatomy, and ending with more clinically relevant information. Typical buzzwords are bolded throughout each chapter to help students remember and associate those commonly used terms. Tables help the reader organize and consolidate information. Similar to **HARDCORE** *Pharmacology*, commonly tested neuroscience principles and critical concepts have been singled out into hardcore boxes for rapid review throughout the text—if you remember nothing else from your studies, remember those!

The book has been organized by systems to closely represent the contents tested in Step 1, with special chapters devoted to clinical correlates (Hardcore Clinical Topics) and commonly encountered imaging findings (Hardcore Imaging). A chapter containing 25 Q&As in the current board format allows for integration of the information and additional Step 1 practice.

The **HARDCORE** series is for students taking Step 1, written by students who have recently taken Step 1, and **HARDCORE** *Neuroscience* is designed for students with limited time to review the most critical concepts of neuroanatomy and medical neuroscience often tested on USMLE Step 1. We believe this is one of the most hardcore, high-yield, yet comprehensive neuroscience review books available, and we hope that you find this text useful and welcome your feedback. Best of luck in your medical journey.

Kevin C. Wang
Rita A. Mukhtar

Reviewers

Neil Patel
Class of 2006
UCLA David Geffen School of Medicine
Los Angeles, California

Serge Hougier
Class of 2006
University of Arizona College of Medicine
Phoenix, Arizona

Adam Kotowski
Class of 2006
SUNY Buffalo School of Medicine and Biomedical Sciences
Buffalo, New York

Dante Maria Chase Foster
Class of 2006
Harvard Medical School
Boston, Massachusetts

Alexander Tsai
Class of 2006
Case Western Reserve University
Cleveland, Ohio

Fatima Cody Stanford
Class of 2006
Medical College of Georgia School of Medicine
Augusta, Georgia

Jamie Hess
Class of 2006
Mayo Medical School
Rochester, Minnesota

Acknowledgments

This book is a product of efforts and contributions from a lot of important players. Many thanks to Beverly Copland, Ben Sears, and Rodrigo Saenz for introducing us to the idea of the Hardcore Series and for allowing us to participate in making this book a reality. A big thank-you goes to Kate Heinle for her assistance with seemingly every single aspect of the project and for being so patient, enthusiastic, positive, and flexible with the production of the manuscript. The contributions from the student reviewers were instrumental in shaping the book into its final form—their insight and feedback are much appreciated. Finally, this book is dedicated to our families, whose support, love, and understanding helped carry us through the entire process.

Kevin C. Wang
Rita A. Mukhtar

Table of Contents

About the Authors / vi
A Note to the Reader / vii
Reviewers / ix
Acknowledgments / xi

1 Cellular Neurophysiology 1

Neurons / 1
Glial Cells / 1
Neural Signaling / 2

2 Synapses and Neurotransmitters 5

Types of Synapses / 5
Neurotransmitters and Their Receptors / 5
Neuromuscular Junction / 6

3 Development and Embryology 7

Neural Plate / 7
Neural Tube / 9
Congenital Infections / 10

4 Gross Anatomy 11

Cerebral Vasculature / 11
Cerebrum / 12
Diencephalon/Midbrain / 14

5 Brainstem Anatomy 17

Structure of the Brainstem / 17
Vertebrobasilar System / 21

6 Cranial Nerves 23

Structure and Function of the Cranial Nerves / 23

7 Spinal Cord and Peripheral Nerves 29

Gross Anatomy / 29
Important Tracts of the Spinal Cord / 31
Spinal Reflexes / 32
Upper and Lower Motor Neuron Syndromes / 33
Classic Spinal Cord Syndromes / 34
Peripheral Nerve Disorders / 34

8 Autonomic Nervous System 37

Organization of the Autonomic Nervous System / 37
Receptors and Pharmacology of the ANS / 40
Enteric Nervous System / 42
Autonomic Control / 42

9 Sensory Systems 43

Sensory Receptors / 43
Ascending Tracts of the Spinal Cord / 43
Pathologic States of the Somatosensory System / 47

10 Motor Systems 49

Cortical Motor Areas / 49

Brainstem Motor Areas / 50
Descending Tracts of the Spinal Cord / 50
The Cerebellum and Basal Ganglia / 51

11 Higher Functions and the Limbic System...**55**

Basic Anatomy and Major Structures / 55
Types of Memory / 58

12 Paroxysmal Disorders..**59**

Seizures / 59
Headaches / 61
Sleep Disorders / 62

13 Cerebrospinal Fluid and Central Nervous System Infections.........**63**

Meninges / 63
Lumbar Puncture / 63
Ventricular System / 64
Infections of the Central Nervous System / 64

14 Space-Occupying Lesions..**67**

Intracranial Compartments and Increased Intracranial Pressure (ICP) / 67
Brain Tumors / 67
Intracranial Bleeds / 69

15 Hardcore Clinical Topics...**71**

Myopathic Disorders / 71
Disorders of Equilibrium / 72
Dementia / 73
Cerebrovascular Disease / 74

16 Hardcore Imaging...**77**

Plain X-Rays / 77
Computerized Axial Tomography / 77
Magnetic Resonance Imaging / 78
Angiography / 79
Images / 80

17 Step 1 Practice Questions and Answers.......................................**85**

Index / 97

CHAPTER 1

Cellular Neurophysiology

The nervous system must transmit information rapidly over long distances. To do this, neurons actively generate electrical signals called action potentials that quickly travel along long, thin fibers which connect each neuron with its target. There are two main types of cells in the nervous system: nerve cells (neurons) and glial cells. These cells have special properties that allow them to carry out their respective signaling and supportive functions.

NEURONS

Properties of Neurons
Neurons differ from other cells of the body in that:

- *They are polarized* to allow for directionality of impulse transmission
- *They are electrically and chemically excitable*
- Their cell bodies contain proteins/organelles for *secretion of signaling molecules (neurotransmitters)*

Structure of Neurons
- Cell body—Contains nucleus
- Dendrites—Short processes that branch out from cell body and receive information for excitation or inhibition
- <u>A</u>xon—Long tubular structure that conducts signal <u>a</u>way from the cell body

Types of Neurons
Neurons can be classified on the basis of the number, length, and mode of branching of their processes:

- Unipolar (e.g., dorsal root ganglion)
- Bipolar (e.g., retinal bipolar cells)
- Multipolar (e.g., neurons in brain and spinal cord)

GLIAL CELLS

Microglia
- Derived from phagocytes and activated during infections, injuries, and seizures
- Equivalent to brain macrophages
- Have CD4 receptors (and are thus susceptible to infection by HIV)

Macroglia
- Oligodendrocytes
- Schwann cells
- Astrocytes

The CNS contains 10–50 times more glia than neurons, and they act to:

- Surround cell bodies, axons, and dendrites of neurons
- Scavenge debris after neuronal injury or cell death
- Contribute to formation of blood-brain barrier
- Myelinate neurons

HARDCORE

Oligodendrocytes:
- *Found in central nervous system (CNS)*
- Each oligodendrocyte myelinates multiple neurons

HARDCORE

Schwann cells:
- *Found in peripheral nervous system (PNS)*
- Up to 500 Schwann cells myelinate a single peripheral neuron
- Spaces in between Schwann cells are called *nodes of Ranvier*

HARDCORE

Astrocytes:
- Most numerous of glial cells
- Irregular, star-shaped borders
- "End-feet" form tight junctions on blood vessels, creating the blood-brain barrier
- Involved in regulation of extracellular ion concentrations, especially K^+

HARDCORE

The myelin sheath is composed of concentric layers of lipids with high cholesterol and phospholipid content. Myelination speeds transmission of action potentials by increasing resistance across the axon membrane.

HARDCORE

One of the most common neurologic disorders, multiple sclerosis (MS) results in scattered areas of *demyelination* in the white matter or the brain and spinal cord, and the optic nerve. Thought to have autoimmune etiology. Associated with:
- *Female gender*
- *Age of onset typically 20–40 years*
- *HLA DR2 antigen*
- Signs and symptoms:
  - *Focal weakness, numbness, tingling*
  - *Blurring and diplopia (due to optic neuritis), or sudden vision loss (due to central scotoma)*
  - *Urinary urgency or hesitancy/retention*
  - *Disequilibrium*
  - *Remitting/relapsing course, often progressive*
  - *Number of lesions on brain scan doesn't necessarily correlate with disease severity*
  - *Increased protein (IgG) in cerebrospinal fluid (oligoclonal bands)*

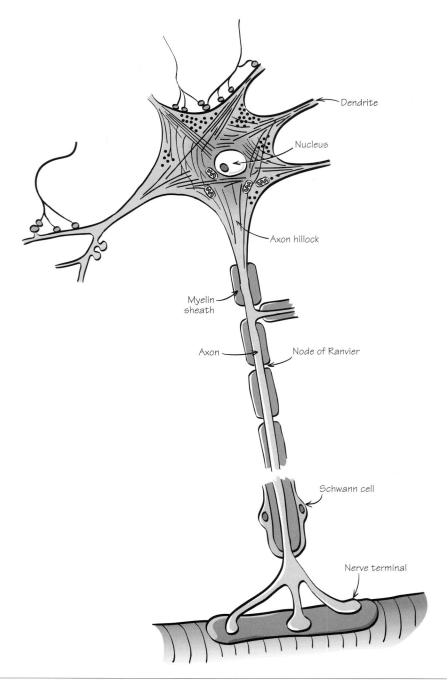

Figure 1-1 Image of basic neuron. Neurons have a cell body, dendrites for receiving information, and an axon for sending information away from the cell body. Note the myelin sheath, which allows for quicker conduction, and the areas that are not myelinated (nodes of Ranvier), at which saltatory conduction occurs. (Modified with permission from Barker RA. Neuroscience at a Glance. 2nd ed. Oxford: Blackwell Publishing, 2003:14.)

NEURAL SIGNALING

- Signaling depends on the electrical properties of the nerve cell membrane
- *Electrical potential* across the cell membrane (*membrane potential*) results from different concentrations of ions inside and outside the cell
- Specific *ion channels* or *ATP-dependent pumps* allow for movement of ions

Ion Channels

- *Voltage-gated*: Open or close depending on the membrane potential
- *Ligand-gated*: Open or close depending on the binding of specific chemical transmitters

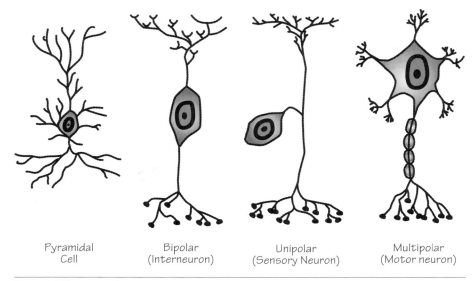

Figure 1-2 Different types of neurons. Neurons come in many shapes and sizes to allow for their specific functions.

Membrane Potential

Membrane potential depends on two factors:

- Electrical potential difference across the membrane
- Concentration gradient of ions across the membrane

Nernst Equation

- Equilibrium potential (E_x) is the membrane potential at which the electrical gradient balances the ion's concentration gradient, and net ion movement is 0
- Each ion strives to bring the membrane potential to its E_x
- More-permeating ions contribute more to the overall membrane potential
- Nernst equation allows calculation of any ion's E_x

$$E_x = (RT/zF) \ln([X \text{ outside}]/[X \text{ inside}])$$

R = Gas constant
T = Temperature (in Kelvin)
z = Valence of ion (+ for cations, – for anions)
F = Faraday constant
X = Concentration of the ion in question

For monovalent ions (z = ±1) near room temperature, this can be simplified to:

$$E_x = \pm 60 \log([X \text{ outside}]/[X \text{ inside}])$$

HARDCORE

Sodium-potassium ATPase (Na^+/K^+-ATPase): ATP-dependent pump that moves K^+ into cells and Na^+ out of cells. Remember "*pump-K-in*" (three Na^+ ions out for every two K^+ ions in).
- Essential for maintaining ionic gradient
- Excess positive charge outside the cell makes the inside relatively negative
- Resting potential of neurons: −60 to −70 mV

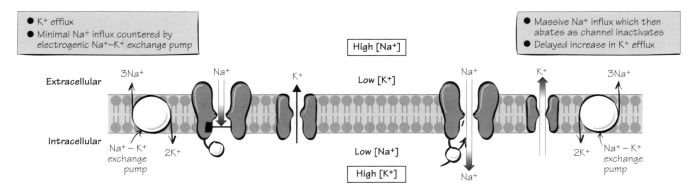

Figure 1-3 Resting potential of neurons. The sodium-potassium pump uses ATP to transport more positive ions outward than inward, making a direct contribution of several millivolts to the membrane potential. (Reprinted with permission from Barker RA. Neuroscience at a Glance. 2nd ed. Oxford: Blackwell Publishing, 2003:20.)

Action Potential

Neural signaling depends on the generation of an "*action potential*," which results from depolarization of the membrane.

- *Depolarization*: Decreased negativity of the membrane potential (closer to zero)
- *Hyperpolarization*: Increased negativity of the membrane potential (farther from zero)

Characteristics of Action Potentials

- Triggered by *depolarization* to *threshold membrane potential*
- *All-or-none events*
- *Propagate without decrement along axons* via the longitudinal spread of current
- At peak, membrane potential reverses and becomes positive
- Cell repolarizes as positive charge leaves
- Immediately after spike of the action potential, the neuron is either unexcitable (*absolute refractory period*) or excitable only by suprathreshold stimuli (*relative refractory period*)

HARDCORE

Many local anesthetics, such as procaine, lidocaine, tetracaine, and cocaine, act by *blocking voltage-dependent Na⁺ channels*, preventing the generation of action potentials. Injection of a local anesthetic near a peripheral nerve blocks action potentials in all sensory and motor fibers within the nerve, producing loss of sensation and paralysis. Naturally occurring biological toxins such as tetrodotoxin (TTX) from puffer fish act similarly.

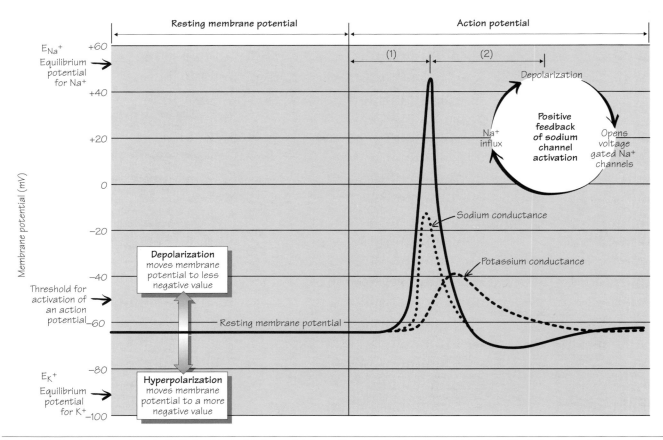

Figure 1-4 The four states of an action potential. Resting state, depolarization, repolarization, and hyperpolarization. During hyperpolarization, the cell is refractory to generation of new action potentials. Conductance depends on permeability to that particular ion. (Modified with permission from Barker RA. Neuroscience at a Glance. 2nd ed. Oxford: Blackwell Publishing, 2003:20.)

CHAPTER 2.

Synapses and Neurotransmitters

Synapses are points of contact between nerve cells and their targets where signals are passed from one cell to the next. Synapses can occur between neurons, or between motor neurons and muscle cells at neuromuscular junctions. Signaling can be either electrical, via action potentials, or chemical, via neurotransmitters. Synapses between neurons can be either excitatory or inhibitory.

TYPES OF SYNAPSES

Electrical Synapses

- Cells are connected by **gap junctions**, at which their cytoplasm is continuous
- Current flows directly from one cell to the next

Chemical Synapses

- Cells are separated by synaptic cleft
- Presynaptic neurons have synaptic vesicles containing neurotransmitters
- Presynaptic action potential results in entry of calcium through voltage-gated Ca^{2+} channels
- Rise in intracellular calcium leads to fusion of vesicles with active zone of presynaptic membrane, releasing them into the synaptic cleft (**exocytosis**)
- Neurotransmitters diffuse across the cleft and bind to receptors on the postsynaptic cell membrane
- Neurotransmitters and synaptic vesicle membranes are recycled through **endocytosis** by presynaptic neurons

NEUROTRANSMITTERS AND THEIR RECEPTORS

Different neurons utilize different molecules as neurotransmitters.

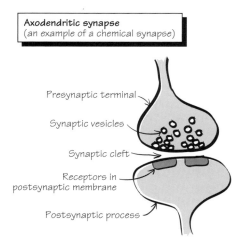

Axodendritic synapse
(an example of a chemical synapse)

Presynaptic terminal

Synaptic vesicles

Synaptic cleft

Receptors in postsynaptic membrane

Postsynaptic process

Figure 2-1 Chemical synapse. Neurotransmitters released by the presynaptic neuron diffuse across the synaptic cleft and bind receptors on the postsynaptic cell. (Modified with permission from Barker RA. Neuroscience at a Glance. 2nd ed. Oxford: Blackwell Publishing, 2003:14.)

TABLE 2-1	Excitatory Neurotransmitters
EXCITATORY NEUROTRANSMITTERS	**PROPERTIES**
Acetylcholine	• Used for signaling by "*cholinergic*" neurons (in the autonomic nervous system, *all preganglionic neurons*, as well as parasympathetic *postganglionic neurons*, signal with acetylcholine) • Used at *neuromuscular junction* • Bind muscarinic and nicotinic receptors • Degraded by *acetylcholinesterase*
Dopamine	• Binds D1 and D2 receptors • Synthesized from tyrosine • Four major tracts use dopamine, three of which are in the substantia nigra and are involved in *Parkinson's disease* and other movement disorders
Norepinephrine/Epinephrine	• Used by "*adrenergic*" neurons in sympathetic nervous system (see Chapter 8, Autonomic Nervous System) • Synthesized from dopamine
Serotonin	• Binds 5-HT receptors • Implicated in depressive and anxiety disorders
Glutamate	• Most common neurotransmitter in the brain • Binds N-methyl-D-aspartate (NMDA) receptors • Always excitatory; glutamate excitotoxicity has been implicated as important cause of ischemic, anoxic, epileptic, and traumatic neuronal damage

HARDCORE

Benzodiazepines exert their calming effect on the nervous system by increasing the *frequency* of GABA-binding chloride channel opening, thus potentiating the inhibitory effects of GABA. *Barbiturates* increase the *duration* of channel opening, resulting in the same effect.

HARDCORE

Myasthenia gravis is an autoimmune disease in which antibodies are produced against the nicotinic acetylcholine receptor, resulting in fewer functional receptors and muscle weakness.

• Weakness usually involves muscles of eyelid (*ptosis*) and oropharynx (resulting in *dysphagia*)
• Weakness waxes and wanes
• Reversible by drugs that inhibit acetylcholinesterase (neostigmine or edrophonium)
• Associated with thymus pathology (hyperplasia, atrophy, or *thymoma*)

• Inhibitory neurotransmitters include gamma-aminobutyric acid (GABA) and glycine (found primarily in spinal cord)

NEUROMUSCULAR JUNCTION

• Junction between motor neuron and skeletal muscle at specialized regions of muscle membrane called end plates
• Acetylcholine release results in rapid depolarization of muscle end plate
• This depolarization results in activation of voltage-gated Na^+ channels, which converts the end plate potential into an action potential

TABLE 2-2	Differences Between Nervous System Synapses and Neuromuscular Junction	
NEURON-NEURON SYNAPSE	**NEUROMUSCULAR JUNCTION**	
Synapses can be either excitatory or inhibitory	Synapses are excitatory	
Use many different neurotransmitters	Use acetylcholine	
One neuron can receive synaptic input from many different neurons	Each skeletal muscle cell receives input from only one neuron	
Single presynaptic action potential produces small change in postsynaptic membrane potential	Single presynaptic action potential produces large depolarization of muscle cell and triggers postsynaptic action potential	

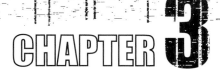

CHAPTER 3

Development and Embryology

The mammalian nervous system develops from a specialized part of the ectoderm, the neural plate. Early on, the embryo is particularly susceptible to genetic and environmental factors that can interfere with normal development. Malformation of the nervous system can result from infections, genetic abnormalities, exposure to toxins, or lack of certain vitamins (e.g., folate) during embryogenesis.

NEURAL PLATE

- Forms during **week 3** of development
- A thickened area of **ectoderm** flanked by **neural crest cells**
- Lateral edges elevate to become neural folds, which join and form the neural tube
- **Open ends of neural tube (neuropores) close during weeks 3–4**

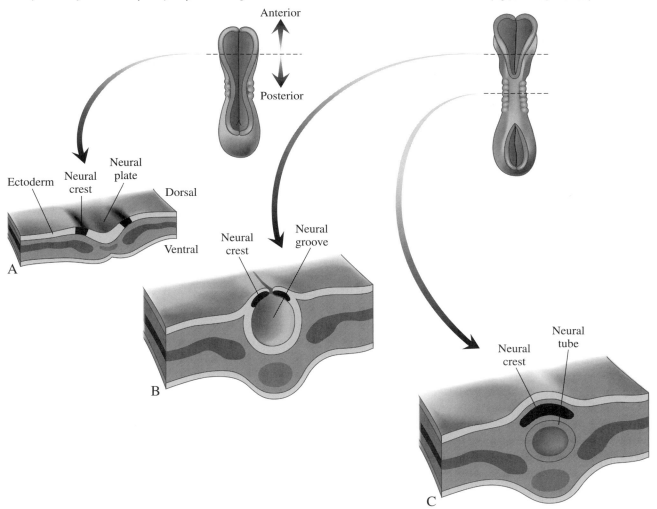

Figure 3-1 Early differentiation of the vertebrate embryonic nervous system. During week 3 of development, ectoderm differentiates into the neural plate. The edges of this plate come together and form the neural tube. (Reprinted with permission from Matthews GG. Neurobiology: Molecules, Cells, Systems. 2nd ed. Malden, MA: Blackwell Publishing, 2001:29.)

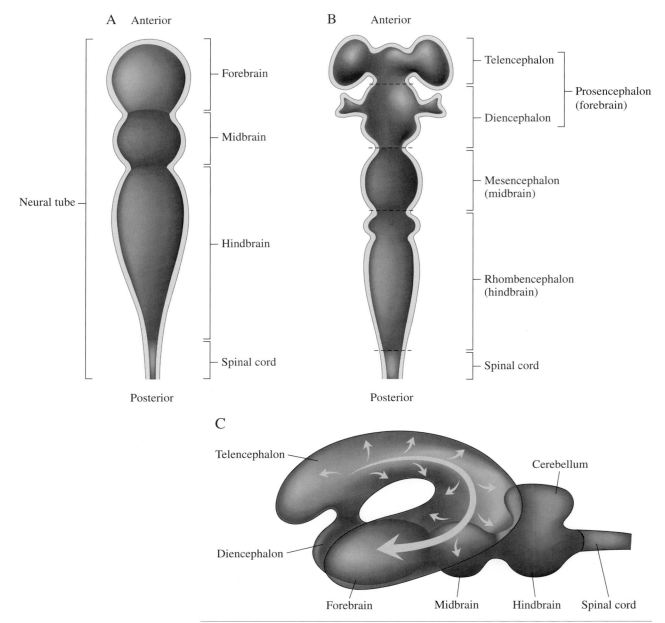

Figure 3-2 Maturation of the brain through development. The three initial dilations (A) of the neural tube undergo further differentiation into their adult derivatives (B and C). (Modified with permission from Matthews GG. Neurobiology: Molecules, Cells, Systems. 2nd ed. Malden, MA: Blackwell Publishing, 2001:30–31.)

NEURAL TUBE

Structures Derived From the Neural Tube

- Cephalic end of neural tube has three dilations representing the primary brain vesicles:
  - ○ *Prosencephalon (forebrain)*
  - ○ *Mesencephalon (midbrain)*
  - ○ *Rhombencephalon (hindbrain)*

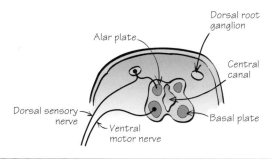

Figure 3-3 Development of the spinal cord. (Modified with permission from Barker RA. Neuroscience at a Glance. 2nd ed. Oxford: Blackwell Publishing, 2003:12.)

- Cells lining the neural tube become **neuroblasts**, or primitive nerve cells, which form both the *gray and the white matter of the spinal cord*

Neural Crest Cells

- Ectodermal in origin
- Appear at lateral edges of neural folds during neural tube development
- Differentiate into:
  - ○ Sympathetic neuroblasts
  - ○ Schwann cells
  - ○ Melanocytes
  - ○ Odontoblasts
  - ○ Meninges (arachnoid and pia)
  - ○ Enteric neurons
  - ○ Dorsal root ganglia
  - ○ Smooth muscle cells

Neural Tube Defects

- Defects can involve meninges, vertebrae, muscles, and skin
- Etiology likely genetic
- Diagnosis:
  - ○ Abnormal ultrasound during pregnancy
  - ○ Elevation in maternal serum or amniotic fluid alpha-fetoprotein level

TABLE 3-1	Characteristics of Various Neural Tube Defects
DISEASE	**CHARACTERISTICS**
Anencephaly	• Lack of brain development
Spina bifida	• Failure of posterior vertebral arches to close; may or may not involve skin
Spina bifida occulta	• Defect in vertebral arches that does not involve skin • Usually in **lumbosacral** region • Overlying skin usually covered by **patch of hair**
Spina bifida cystica	• Neural tissue and/or meninges protrude through defect in vertebral arches and skin • Usually accompanied by **Arnold-Chiari malformation** (herniation of cerebellar structures through foramen magnum)
Meningocele	• Only meninges protrude through defect
Meningomyelocele	• Meninges and neural tissue protrude through defect

HARDCORE

- *Alar plate* of neural tube forms *sensory neurons*
- *Basal plate* of neural tube forms *motor neurons*

HARDCORE

In **Hirschsprung's disease (congenital megacolon)**, failure of neural crest cells to migrate results in the absence of parasympathetic ganglia in all or part of the colon and rectum wall. Most familial cases are due to mutation in gene essential for crest cell migration. Clinical manifestations include **absence of bowel movement**, and dilated colon above the affected region (rectum and sigmoid colon in 80% of patients).

HARDCORE

- Failure of closure of **anterior neuropore** results in **anencephaly**
- Failure of closure of **posterior neuropore** results in **spina bifida**
- *Periconception folate reduces risk of neural tube defects*

HARDCORE

Elevated alpha-fetoprotein in maternal serum or amniotic fluid is associated with **neural tube defects** such as spina bifida and anencephaly. In contrast, Down's syndrome (trisomy 21) and Edwards' syndrome (trisomy 18) are associated with decreased alpha-fetoprotein.

CONGENITAL INFECTIONS

Many congenital infections have profound effects on the nervous system (Table 3.2).

TABLE 3-2 TORCHeS	
DISEASE	**CHARACTERISTICS AND EFFECTS ON NERVOUS SYSTEM**
Toxoplasmosis	• Mental retardation • Seizures • Spasticity • Cerebral calcifications
Rubella	• Deafness • Retinopathy, cataracts • Congenital heart disease (e.g., patent ductus arteriosus) • Teratogenicity is greatest in first trimester
Cytomegalovirus	• Mental retardation • Sensorineural deafness • Cerebral calcifications • Most common congenital infection (mostly asymptomatic)
Herpes simplex	• Mostly HSV-2 (usually transmitted during vaginal delivery) • Seizures • Encephalitis
Syphilis	• Small for gestational age • Meningitis • Deafness • Deformed teeth • Variable outcomes from benign to fatal

Gross Anatomy

A solid grasp of the main anatomic features of the nervous system is essential not only for an appreciation of the normal structural-functional relationships, but also for an understanding of possible mechanisms underlying pathologic disease states.

CEREBRAL VASCULATURE

- Brain contains 98% of the body's neural tissue, weighing about 3 lb
- *Glucose* supplies more than 95% of energy (fat cannot cross blood-brain barrier); *ketone bodies* can cross blood-brain barrier in diabetic ketoacidosis
- Blood is supplied continuously through two main arterial systems:
  - Receives 15% to 20% of total cardiac output at rest
  - *Internal carotid arteries* come up through either side of front of neck
  - *Basilar artery* forms at base of the skull from vertebral arteries
  - Carotids and basilar artery terminate in the *circle of Willis*, located at floor of cranial cavity; loop structure ensures continuous blood supply to brain even if one carotid becomes blocked

HARDCORE

The probability of developing significant degenerative arterial disease (*atherosclerosis* and *lipohyalinosis*) is increased by certain risk factors:

- Smoking
- Hypertension
- Diabetes mellitus
- Hypercholesterolemia
- Family history of vascular disease/stroke
- Age
- Oral contraceptives (secondary to hyper-coagulable state)

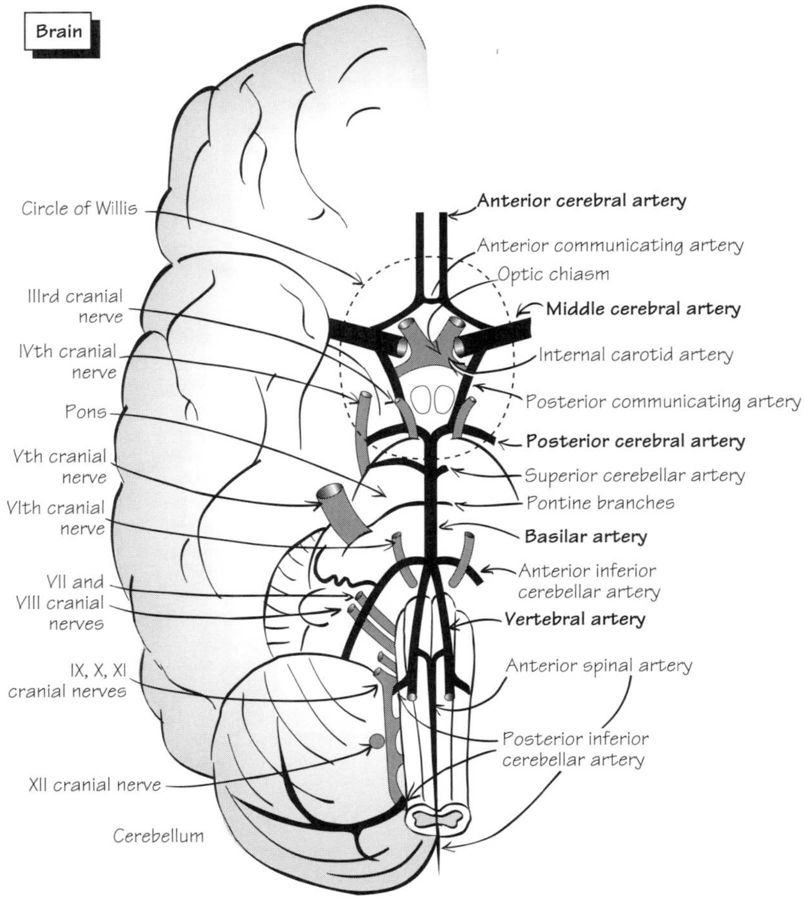

Figure 4-1 **Blood supply to the brain**, demonstrating the vertebrobasilar and carotid arterial systems, showing their course and communication through the circle of Willis. The basilar artery gives off the superior cerebellar arteries before terminating as the posterior cerebral arteries to supply medial portions of the temporal lobes and occipital cortex. Selected cranial nerve exits are also shown. (Modified with permission from Barker RA. Neuroscience at a Glance. 2nd ed. Oxford: Blackwell Publishing, 2003:42.)

HARDCORE

Because cerebral vessels have no anatomic reserves, any obstruction is likely to result in tissue damage. The most common cause is *atherosclerosis*. A stroke is usually defined as one of two types: *Ischemic* (caused by blockage in an artery) or *hemorrhagic* (caused by tear in arterial wall that produces bleeding in the brain). Signs and symptoms of arterial infarcts depend on the vascular territory affected (Figure 4.2):

- *Total anterior (carotid) circulation infarct*: Hemiplegia, hemianopia, and cortical deficits (dysphasia, visual-spatial loss)

- *Lacunar infarct*: Intrinsic disease in small, deep/perforating arteries (*lenticulostriates*) produces characteristic syndrome of pure motor, pure sensory, mixed sensorimotor, or ataxic hemiparesis

- *Posterior/vertebrobasilar circulation infarct*: Vertigo, diplopia, altered consciousness (brainstem lesions), and homonymous hemianopia (with macular sparing)

○ Circle of Willis loops around brainstem above pons, giving off major vessels supplying the brain: The *anterior*, *middle*, and *posterior cerebral arteries*, and the *anterior inferior cerebellar artery* (*AICA*), *posterior inferior cerebellar artery* (*PICA*), *superior cerebellar*, *pontine*, *and labyrinthine branches*

○ Collateral flow partially compensates for damage to single arteries

○ Baroreceptors sense blood pressure in internal carotids (*carotid bulb*)

CEREBRUM

The two cerebral hemispheres are joined together by the *corpus callosum* and *anterior commissure*, and the *longitudinal fissure* divides the cerebrum into left and right hemispheres. The left hemisphere is often dominant. The cerebrum consists of gray (cell bodies of neurons) and white (collection of axons) matter. The hemispheres have lateral and medial surfaces and frontal, temporal, and occipital poles. The surfaces are enfolded forming *gyri* (convexities/folds), *sulci* (valleys), and *fissures* (deeper valleys).

Lateral Surface

- Divided into lobes by sulci and fissures
- Principal sulci are *central sulcus*, dividing the frontal from the parietal lobes, and *lateral (Sylvian) fissure*, which divides the temporal lobe from the frontoparietal lobes
- *Precentral gyrus is motor; postcentral gyrus is sensory*

Medial Surface

- Made up of medial extensions of the frontal, parietal, temporal, and occipital lobes
- Gyri of limbic system form a central ring of cortex bordering the corpus callosum and rostral parts of brainstem
- *Cingulate gyrus* lies just above *corpus callosum* and is separated from frontal lobe and anterior parts of parietal lobe by cingulate sulcus
- *Parieto-occipital sulcus* forms border between parietal and occipital lobes
- *Calcarine sulcus* is a landmark for the primary visual cortex

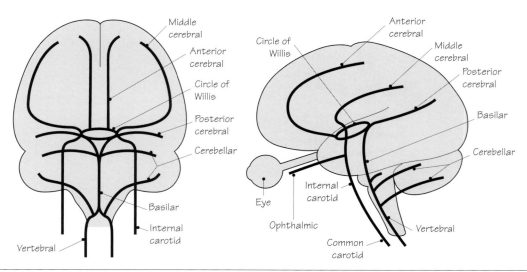

Figure 4-2 Distribution of the anterior, middle, and posterior cerebral arteries. The anterior/carotid circulation consists of anterior and middle cerebral arteries, whereas the posterior circulation is posterior cerebral artery plus branches supplying the brainstem and cerebellum. (Reprinted with permission from Wilkinson I. Essential Neurology. 4th ed. Oxford: Blackwell Publishing, 2005:27.)

Functional Lobes

Frontal Lobe

- *Precentral gyrus* is location of primary motor cortex
- Representation of *Broca's speech area*, which is responsible for expressive speech (usually in left hemisphere)

Temporal Lobe

- The primary cortical area for auditory input is located on *superior temporal gyrus* buried within lateral fissure
- *Wernicke's speech area*, which is responsible for understanding speech, is located posterior to junction of temporal and parietal lobes (usually in left hemisphere)

Parietal Lobe

- *Postcentral gyrus* is the primary cortical area receiving somatosensory input from the body and head
- Also somatotopically organized in mediolateral direction

Occipital Lobe

- Visual processing

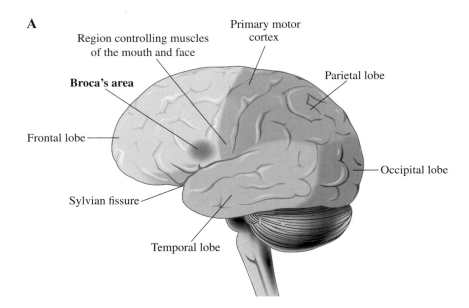

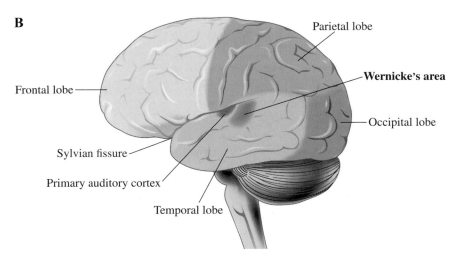

Figure 4-3 Lobes of the cerebral cortex with locations of Broca's (A) and Wernicke's (B) areas, in the frontal and temporal lobes of the left hemisphere, respectively. Lesions in Broca's interfere with production of spoken language (**expressive aphasia**), while lesions in Wernicke's interfere with comprehension of spoken language (**receptive aphasia**). (Reprinted with permission from Matthews GG. Neurobiology: Molecules, Cells, Systems. 2nd ed. Malden, MA: Blackwell Publishing, 2001:500−501.)

Internal Capsule

- Large white matter axons projecting to and from cerebral cortex
- Anterior limb divides the *caudate* and *putamen* nuclei; the posterior limb passes between *thalamus* and *globus pallidus*

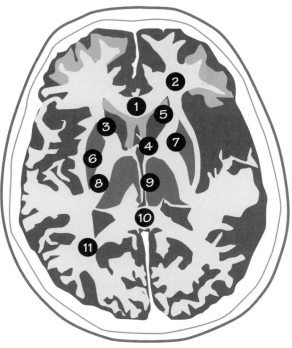

1. Genu of corpus callosum
2. Forceps minor
3. Anterior limb of internal capsule
4. Septum pellucidum
5. Caudate nucleus
6. Putamen
7. Globus pallidus
8. Posterior limb of internal capsule
9. Thalamus
10. Splenium of corpus callosum
11. Forceps major

Figure 4-4 Schematic of a transverse MRI of the brain at the level of the internal capsule.

Lateral Ventricles

- C-shaped ventricular cavities in each hemisphere
- Each divided into anterior horn (associated with frontal lobe), posterior horn (deep to occipital lobe), and inferior horn (in temporal lobe)
- *Septum pellucidum* separates anterior horns

DIENCEPHALON/MIDBRAIN

Thalamus

- Dorsal thalamus is an egg-shaped mass of nuclei that project topographically to cerebral cortex
- Relays visual, auditory, somatosensory, motor, and multimodal information
- Bordered laterally by internal capsule and medially by third ventricle

Hypothalamus

- Small region containing nuclei associated with limbic and vegetative functions (appetite, thirst, temperature regulation, sex, and aggression)
- Located ventral and rostral to the thalamus; caudal boundary marked by mammillary bodies
- Stalk of the pituitary (infundibulum) arises from ventral surface of hypothalamus; hypothalamic neurons exert much of their influence by neuronal and vascular signals to the pituitary

Third Ventricle

- Forms a narrow slit between the thalami and hypothalami
- Communicates with lateral ventricles by *interventricular foramen (of Monro)*
- Forms two recesses above the optic tract and infundibulum

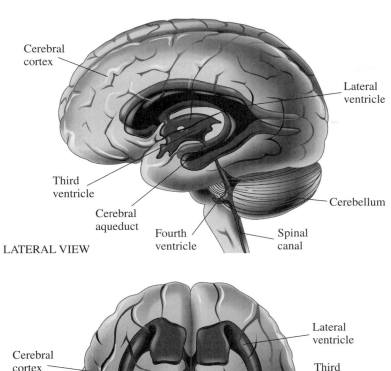

LATERAL VIEW

ANTERIOR VIEW

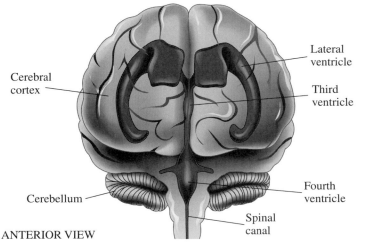

Figure 4-5 Lateral and anterior views of the ventricles of the brain. (Reprinted with permission from Matthews GG. Neurobiology: Molecules, Cells, Systems. 2nd ed. Malden, MA: Blackwell Publishing, 2001:33.)

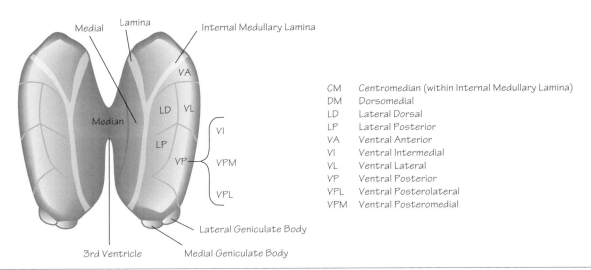

CM	Centromedian (within Internal Medullary Lamina)
DM	Dorsomedial
LD	Lateral Dorsal
LP	Lateral Posterior
VA	Ventral Anterior
VI	Ventral Intermedial
VL	Ventral Lateral
VP	Ventral Posterior
VPL	Ventral Posterolateral
VPM	Ventral Posteromedial

Figure 4-6 Schematic representation of the thalamus. The thalamus serves as a sensory relay station for all somatic, auditory, and visual input to the cerebral cortex. A few of the named nuclei have clinically significant roles.

TABLE 4-1	Thalamic Nuclei and Their Functions		
NUCLEUS	INPUT	OUTPUT	FUNCTION
Anterior	Mammillothalamic tract	Cingulate gyrus	Limbic and memory
Ventral anterior	Basal ganglia	Premotor cortex	Motor
Ventral lateral	Dentate nucleus	Motor and premotor cortices	Motor
Ventral posterior lateral	Dorsal column system	Postcentral gyrus	Somatosensory (body)
Ventral posterior medial	Trigeminal system	Postcentral gyrus	Somatosensory (face)
Lateral geniculate	Retina	Visual cortex	Vision
Medial geniculate	Inferior colliculus	Auditory cortex	Hearing
Dorsomedial	Amygdala	Prefrontal cortex	Limbic and memory
Centromedian	Reticular formation	Multiple cortical areas	Reticular activating system

(Modified with permission from Wechsler RT. Blueprints Notes & Cases: Neuroscience. Malden, MA: Blackwell Publishing, 2004:49.)

Tectum

- Forms roof of cerebral aqueduct, the ventricular cavity of the midbrain
- Consists of superior and inferior colliculi, which function in reflexive movements of the head and eyes to sudden auditory and visual stimuli, respectively

Tegmentum

- Ventral to the cerebral aqueduct
- Contains cranial nerve nuclei III and IV, red nucleus, and substantia nigra
- Reticular formation located in the core of midbrain tegmentum

Cerebral Peduncles

- Located in the most ventral part of the midbrain
- Contain axons whose cell bodies are located in the precentral gyrus

For information on the main anatomical features of the brainstem and the cerebellum, see Chapter 5, Brainstem Anatomy, and Chapter 10, Motor Systems, respectively.

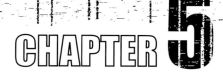

CHAPTER 5

Brainstem Anatomy

The brainstem extends from the pyramidal decussation to the posterior commissure. This part of the brain is essential for survival: Not only does the brainstem serve as a processing site for sensory information that passes from the spinal cord to the forebrain, it contains structures essential for maintaining basic functions, e.g., breathing and consciousness. Additionally, the cranial nerves have their origin in the brainstem.

STRUCTURE OF THE BRAINSTEM

- The CNS can be grossly divided into "brain" and "spinal cord"
- The brain itself is divided into forebrain, midbrain, and hindbrain
- The midbrain and hindbrain together are called the "brainstem"
- The hindbrain has three principal subdivisions:
  - *Pons*
  - *Medulla oblongata*
  - *Cerebellum*

Cranial Nerves

- Cranial nerves (CNs) III–XII are found in the brainstem (except the spinal part of CN XI)
- All CNs (except trochlear, CN IV) exit from the ventral surface of brainstem

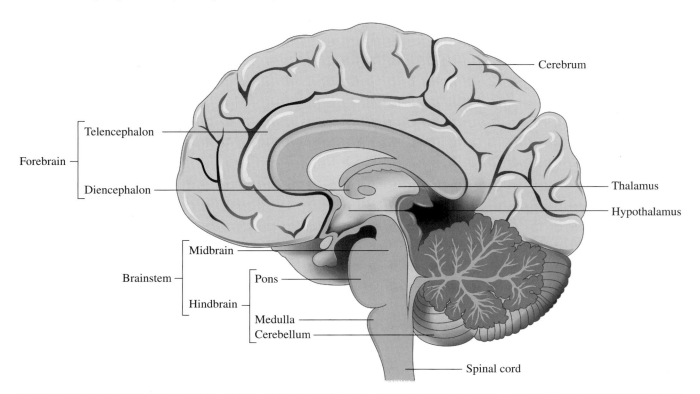

Figure 5-1 Midline sagittal view showing overall structural organization of human brain. The hindbrain is further divided into the pons, medulla, and cerebellum. (Reprinted with permission from Matthews GG. Neurobiology: Molecules, Cells, Systems. 2nd ed. Malden, MA: Blackwell Publishing, 2001:27.)

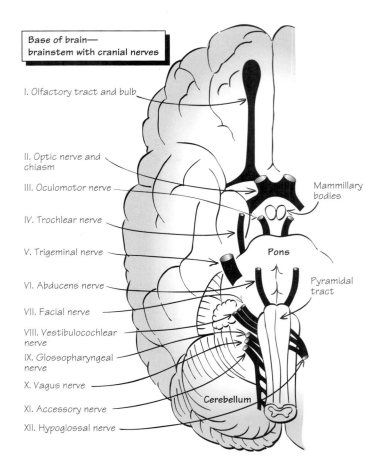

Base of brain—
brainstem with cranial nerves

I. Olfactory tract and bulb

II. Optic nerve and chiasm

III. Oculomotor nerve

IV. Trochlear nerve

V. Trigeminal nerve

VI. Abducens nerve

VII. Facial nerve

VIII. Vestibulocochlear nerve

IX. Glossopharyngeal nerve

X. Vagus nerve

XI. Accessory nerve

XII. Hypoglossal nerve

Mammillary bodies

Pons

Pyramidal tract

Cerebellum

Figure 5-2 Ventral surface of brainstem with cranial nerves emerging. CNs III and IV exit superior to the pons; V exits from the pons; VI, VII, and VIII exit between the pons and medulla; and IX, X, XI, and XII emerge from the medulla. (Modified with permission from Barker RA. Neuroscience at a Glance. 2nd ed. Oxford: Blackwell Publishing, 2003:36.)

- Sections through brainstem reveal **nuclei of cranial nerves**, and **tracts of motor and sensory fibers** running through brainstem

Structures of the Midbrain

- **Nuclei of CN III**: Edinger-Westphal, oculomotor
- **Nucleus of CN IV**: Trochlear nucleus
  - Fibers of trochlear nerve exit dorsally, cross midline, and head toward orbits
- Red nucleus, substantia nigra, cerebral peduncles (paramedian structures) (predominantly motor function)
- **Medial lemniscus and spinothalamic tracts**: Main sensory pathways traveling through midbrain
- **Periaqueductal gray matter**: Contains nuclei involved in **analgesia**; surrounds cerebral aqueduct

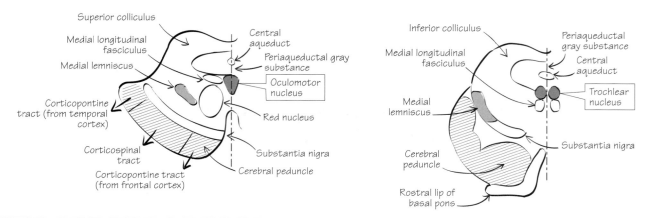

Figure 5-3 Axial sections of upper and lower midbrain. (Reprinted with permission from Barker RA. Neuroscience at a Glance. 2nd ed. Oxford: Blackwell Publishing, 2003:36.)

Structures of the Pons

- *Nuclei of CN V*: Trigeminal sensory nucleus and trigeminal motor nucleus
- *Nucleus of CN VI*: Abducens nucleus
- *Nucleus of CN VII*: Facial nerve
- *Nucleus of CN VIII*: Vestibulocochlear nerve
- Medial longitudinal fasciculus (MLF)

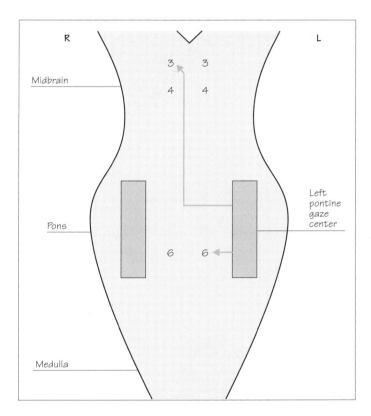

HARDCORE

Normal lateral gaze requires synchronous contraction of the lateral rectus muscle (controlled by CN VI) of one eye, and medial rectus (controlled by CN III) of the other. CN III is activated in response to CN VI via the *medial longitudinal fasciculus (MLF)*. Damage to the MLF results in failure of medial gaze on the ipsilateral side during attempted lateral gaze. Convergence is unaffected. Most commonly seen in *multiple sclerosis*.

Figure 5-4 Internuclear ophthalmoplegia (INO). (Reprinted with permission from Wilkinson I Essential Neurology. 4th ed. Oxford: Blackwell Publishing, 2005:27.)

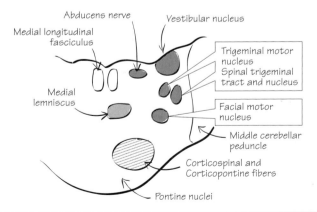

Figure 5-5 Cross-section of midpons. (Reprinted with permission from Barker RA. Neuroscience at a Glance. 2nd ed. Oxford: Blackwell Publishing, 2003:34.)

Structures of the Medulla

Pyramids
- Longitudinally arranged fascicles visible on ventral surface
- Contain axons of *corticospinal tract*
- Fibers cross at *decussation of pyramids*

Inferior Olives
- Protrusions lateral to pyramids
- Contain inferior olivary nuclei, which project to cerebellum via inferior cerebellar peduncles

Nuclei (of dorsal columns/medial lemniscus system)
- *Nucleus gracilis*: Receives projections of lower thoracic, lumbar, and sacral dorsal root ganglion neurons
- *Nucleus cuneatus*: Receives projections of cervical/upper thoracic dorsal root ganglion neurons
  - These nuclei give rise to arcuate fibers that *cross midline* and form *ascending medial lemniscus*
- Spinothalamic pathway fibers (dorsolateral to pyramidal tract, inferior olivary nuclei, and MLF)
- MLF: Extends from pons through spinal cord
- *Nucleus ambiguous*
  - Origin of motor output for CNs IX, X, and XI
- *Nucleus solitarius*
  - Receives sensory information via CNs IX and X, via tractus solitarius
- Spinal nucleus of trigeminal nerve
- Nucleus of CN XII

HARDCORE

- Disruption of nucleus a**M**biguous impairs **M**otor function to CNs IX, X, and XI
- Results in *hoarseness, dysarthria, and dysphagia*

HARDCORE

Causes of coma:

A = Apoplexy (brainstem infarction, intracranial hemorrhage)

E = Epilepsy (postictal state, interictal state, status epilepticus)

I = Injury (concussion)

I = Infection (cerebral abscess, meningoencephalitis)

O = Opiates (respiratory depression, also alcohol)

U = Uremia (other metabolic causes include anoxia, hypoglycemia, liver failure, carbon dioxide narcosis)

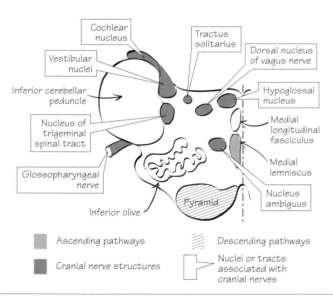

Figure 5-6 Upper medulla in cross section. (Reprinted with permission from Barker RA. Neuroscience at a Glance. 2nd ed. Oxford: Blackwell Publishing, 2003:34.)

Reticular Formation
- Central core of nuclei running through entire length of brainstem
- Controls level of *consciousness, cardiovascular,* and *respiratory systems*
- Contains ascending projections to forebrain essential for consciousness (*reticular activating system*)
- Caudal reticular formation involved in *motor reflexes* and *autonomic functions*
- Raphe nuclei are midline *serotonergic* nuclei involved with *sleep* and *nociception*

VERTEBROBASILAR SYSTEM

- The blood supply to the brainstem

Vertebral Arteries

- Arise from subclavian arteries
- Branches include:
  - ○ *Anterior and posterior spinal arteries*
  - ○ *Posterior inferior cerebellar artery (PICA)*
- *Branches supply dorsolateral quadrant of medulla* containing nucleus ambiguous and CNs IX, X, and XI

Basilar Artery

- Formed by the two vertebral arteries that meet at base of pons

HARDCORE

Occlusion of the basilar artery at the junction of the two PCAs results in *total blindness*, since the PCAs supply the visual cortex.

TABLE 5-1 Branches of the Basilar Artery and Regions Supplied

BRANCH OF BASILAR ARTERY (LISTED FROM CAUDAL TO ROSTRAL DIRECTION)	REGION SUPPLIED
Anterior inferior cerebellar artery (AICA)	Caudal lateral pontine tegmentum (including CN VII), spinal trigeminal tract of CN V, and *inferior surface of cerebellum*
Pontine arteries (paramedian branches)	Base of *pons*, including corticospinal fibers and exiting fibers of CN VI
Superior cerebellar artery (SCA)	Dorsolateral tegmentum of rostral pons, superior cerebellar peduncle, *superior surface of cerebellum and cerebellar nuclei*, and cochlear nuclei
Posterior cerebral artery (PCA)	*Midbrain*, thalamus, and *occipital lobe*

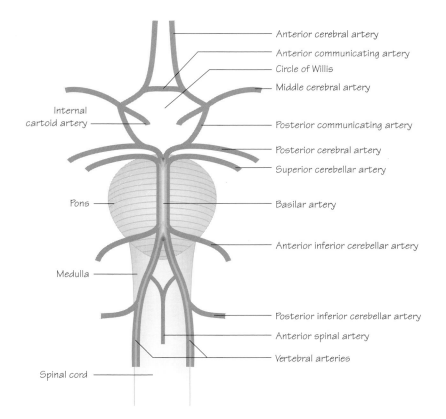

HARDCORE

The circle of Willis, the anastomotic ring at the base of the brain, allows *shunting of blood between the right and left cerebral hemispheres* (via the *anterior communicating artery*), and *between the anterior and posterior systems* (via the *posterior communicating arteries*). These communications are important in patients with occlusion of one of the major cervical arteries.

Figure 5-7 Circle of Willis. (Reprinted with permission from Wechsler RT. Blueprints Notes & Cases: Neuroscience. Malden, MA: Blackwell Publishing, 2004:143.)

CHAPTER 6

Cranial Nerves

The cranial nerves (CNs) serve similar functions in the head and neck as the spinal nerves do for the rest of the body. In addition, they also mediate a number of other specialized functions, including modulation of heart rate and motility of the gastrointestinal tract. The cranial nerves are numbered sequentially, rostral to caudal, from 1 to 12. Some of the nerves are purely motor, others are purely sensory, and still others are both (motor and sensory). As the brainstem is a very complex structure, disease, when it appears, rarely affects a single system.

STRUCTURE AND FUNCTION OF THE CRANIAL NERVES

Mnemonic (to remember the order and names of the cranial nerves): Oh, oh, oh, to touch and feel very good velvet . . . ah heaven!

CN I (Olfactory)

- Mediates olfaction/smell
- Exits through foramina in *cribiform plate*; does not originate in or pass through brainstem
- One of two (along with taste) *uncrossed* sensations
- Causes of *anosmia* (loss of smell) include tumors (meningioma compressing the olfactory bulb) and head injury (anterior cranial fossa fracture)
- Olfactory auras typical prodromal feature of *uncinate epilepsy*

CN II (Optic)

- Formed by axons of retinal ganglion cells; *mediates vision*
- Input from inferior visual field is received by superior retina and transmitted to superior visual cortex, while input from superior visual field is received by inferior retina and transmitted to inferior visual cortex
- Consists of tracts of *diencephalon* (CNS) that project through optic canal
- Project from nasal hemiretina to contralateral *lateral geniculate body (LGN)*, and from temporal hemiretina to ipsilateral LGN
- LGN projects to primary visual cortex via optic radiations; *Meyer's loop* arises from ventral portion of optic tracts to loop anteriorly in temporal lobe
- *Optic chiasm* contains decussating fibers from nasal hemiretinas

CN III (Oculomotor)

- Moves eye, constricts pupil, accommodates, and converges
- Innervates four extraocular muscles and levator palpebrae
- Arises from ipsilateral *oculomotor nucleus* of rostral midbrain
- Enters orbit through *superior orbital fissure*

CN IV (Trochlear)

- Pure motor nerve innervating superior oblique muscle (*remember "SO4"*)
- Arises from contralateral *trochlear nucleus* of caudal midbrain, *crosses midline*
- *Exits brainstem dorsally*, enters orbit through superior orbital fissure
- Palsy results in *vertical diplopia*

CN V (Trigeminal)

- Innervates *muscles of mastication*
- Cutaneous and proprioceptive sensations from face, mouth, and teeth
- Derived from brachial arch 1 (mandibular)
- Arises from trigeminal nuclei in *pontine tegmentum*

HARDCORE

Pituitary adenomas produce two principal sets of symptoms: Space-occupying effects and endocrine disturbance. When the pituitary gland enlarges in its fossa, it commonly expands upward to compress optic nerve/chiasm/tracts, resulting in the classic finding of **bitemporal hemianopsia**. Lateral expansion can compress structures on the lateral wall of cavernous sinus, producing double vision.

HARDCORE

Light shined into one eye causes both pupils to constrict; response of stimulated eye is termed **direct pupillary light reflex**; that of opposite eye is **consensual light reflex**. Lack of direct light reflex is usually due to ipsilateral optic nerve lesion, while lack of consensual light reflex is usually due to a lesion in CN III in the unresponsive eye.

HARDCORE

Transtentorial (uncal) herniation occurs when pressure inside the skull (intracranial pressure) increases and displaces brain tissue. It commonly results from cerebral edema or space-occupying lesions within the brain such as tumors or bleeds. Most commonly, a portion of the **temporal lobe** (**uncus**) is displaced through the tentorial notch, compressing CN III, midbrain, and the posterior cerebral artery. See **fixed and dilated pupil and external strabismus** (exotropia).

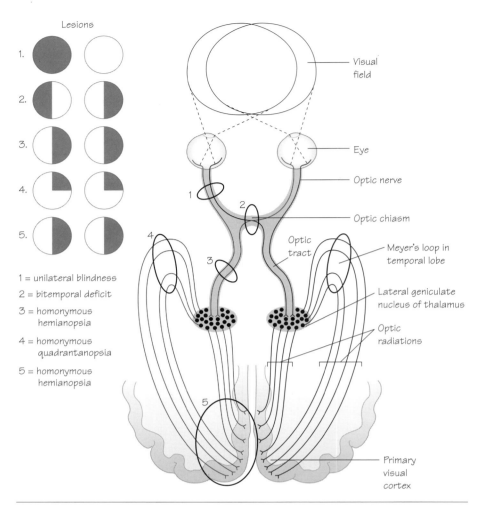

Lesions

1 = unilateral blindness

2 = bitemporal deficit

3 = homonymous
    hemianopsia

4 = homonymous
    quadrantanopsia

5 = homonymous
    hemianopsia

Figure 6-1 Lesions of the visual pathways. Anatomy of the visual pathways with most common types of lesions occurring therein. Diseases of the optic nerve (such as multiple sclerosis) lead to loss of vision in the affected eye (monocular blindness, 1). Compression of optic chiasm by adjacent pituitary tumor leads to bitemporal hemianopsia (2). Vascular and neoplastic lesions of the optic tract, optic radiation, or occipital cortex produce a contralateral homonymous hemianopsia (3 and 5). Temporal lobe lesions involving Meyer's loop result in loss of vision in contralateral upper and outer quadrants (homonymous quadrantanopia, 4). (Reprinted with permission from Wechsler RT. Blueprints Notes & Cases: Neuroscience. Malden, MA: Blackwell Publishing, 2004:98.)

HARDCORE

The pupillary light reflex is a reflex arc containing both afferent (CN II) and efferent limbs (CN III). It includes retinal ganglion cells that project bilaterally to the pretectal nuclei, then to the *Edinger-Westphal nucleus* of CN III. The pathway continues with parasympathetic fibers, synapsing first with neurons of the *ciliary ganglion* then the sphincter muscle of the iris, resulting in pupillary constriction (*miosis*).

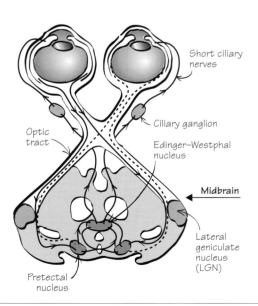

Figure 6-2 Parasympathetic innervation of the pupil and pathway. (Modified with permission from Barker RA. Neuroscience at a Glance. 2nd ed. Oxford: Blackwell Publishing, 2003:34.)

- *Only CN that exits from body of pons*
- Has three branches:
  - V1: *Ophthalmic* exits via *superior orbital fissure*
  - V2: *Maxillary* exits via *foramen rotundum*
  - V3: *Mandibular* exits via *foramen ovale*

CN VI (Abducens)

- Pure motor nerve innervating lateral rectus muscle (*remember "LR6"*)
- Arises from *abducent nucleus* in caudal pons, enters orbit through superior orbital fissure
- Most common isolated palsy seen with subarachnoid hemorrhage, advanced syphilis, meningitis, and trauma
- Palsy results in *horizontal diplopia*

CN VII (Facial)

- Responsible for almost all motor function of face (except opening eyes, which is done by CN III via levator palpebrae superioris)
  - Motor cortex sends signal via *corticobulbar tract*
  - Fibers of corticobulbar tract *cross and synapse at facial nucleus* in pons, where *lower motor neurons continue to innervate upper and lower halves of face*
  - *Each* motor cortex also sends fibers *directly* to *ipsilateral* facial nucleus (without crossing); *lower motor neurons continue only to upper half of face*
  - *Lower half of face* is therefore controlled by *only contralateral motor cortex*
  - *Upper half of face* is controlled by *both contralateral and ipsilateral* motor cortex
- Responsible for cutaneous sensation of external ear (*geniculate ganglion*)
- Gustatory fibers hitchhike on lingual branch of trigeminal nerve to form *chorda tympani*; governs taste of anterior two-thirds of tongue
- Motor: Input to *muscles of facial expression*; lacrimal glands; *salivary glands* (not parotid)
- Derived from brachial arch 2 (hyoid)
- Formed from projections of *facial nucleus* in pons
- Passes through *internal auditory meatus*

HARDCORE

Lesions of the trigeminal nerve include:

- *Herpes zoster* infection of sensory roots of CN V (*shingles*) leads to pain and eruption of vesicles localized to the dermatome supplied by one of its branches. Varicella virus is latent in the trigeminal ganglion.
- *Trigeminal neuralgia* may be most common disease affecting CN V, characterized by attacks of brief, severe, stabbing, electric shock-like jolts pain in the territory of one of more divisions of the nerve. Affects older patients (>50 y). Attributable to aberrant nerve compression by arterial loop.

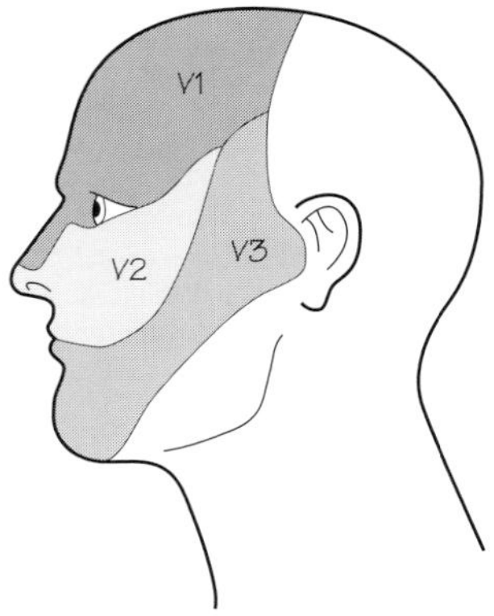

Figure 6-3 Areas of the skin supplied by each branch of the trigeminal nerve. (Reprinted with permission from Wilkinson I. Essential Neurology. 4th ed. Oxford: Blackwell Publishing, 2005:122).

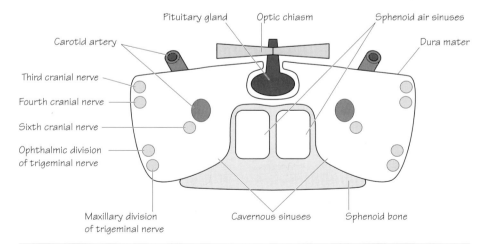

Figure 6-4 Cross-section through cavernous sinus. (Reprinted with permission from Wechsler RT. Blueprints Notes & Cases: Neuroscience. Malden, MA: Blackwell Publishing, 2004:152.)

HARDCORE

- Part of the dural venous sinus system, the cavernous sinuses are lateral to the sphenoid sinuses and connected by venous plexuses
- Contain cranial nerves that pass through *superior orbital fissure*:
  - *CNs III, IV, VI* and *ophthalmic branch of CN V*
- Also contain *maxillary branch of CN V* (passes through *foramen rotundum*)
- Contain *carotid arteries*
- Symptoms of cavernous sinus disease (thrombosis, tumors) can include:
  - Dysfunctional extraocular movement
  - Pupillary abnormalities, proptosis
  - Periorbital inflammation
  - Conjunctival injection
  - Face/head pain

HARDCORE

Bell's palsy is an acute **unilateral lower motor neuron (LMN) lesion** of CN VII within its course through the skull. Symptoms include ear pain, failure of eye closure, absent corneal reflex, hyperacusis on affected side, and loss of sensation in anterior two-thirds of tongue. Thought to be secondary to a viral or postviral phenomenon. Majority of patients recover completely. Severe cases result in tearing of eye with salivation ("**crocodile tears**") from inappropriate regeneration of facial nerve.

HARDCORE

Acoustic neuroma is a **benign tumor** of CN VIII that leads to compression of the nerve and adjacent structures in the **cerebellopontine angle**. Attacks of dizziness are accompanied by profound deafness; expansion of tumor results in ataxia and paralysis of CN V–VIII and the limbs. Unilateral and bilateral acoustic neuromas are found in **neurofibromatosis**.

- Clinical significance:
  - ○ Lesion of **upper motor neuron** of CN VII results in **paralysis of contralateral lower half of face only** (upper half of face still has intact lower motor neuron, receiving input from ipsilateral motor cortex)
  - ○ Lesion of **lower motor neuron** of CN VII (e.g., Bell's palsy) results in **paralysis of entire ipsilateral side** of face (no input from either motor cortex can reach facial muscles)

CN VIII (Vestibulocochlear)

- Two functional divisions—**vestibular** (equilibrium, balance) and **cochlear** (hearing)—that pass through internal auditory meatus
- Static labyrinth controls balance; dynamic labyrinth operates vestibulo-ocular reflexes (**nystagmus**)
- Auditory pathways have **bilateral representation** in the inferior colliculus; unilateral deafness suggests a peripheral, nerve, or nuclear lesion
- Enters brain at junctional region of pons and medulla (**cerebellopontine angle**)
- Deafness can be **conductive** (peripheral disease in outer ear canal or middle ear) or **sensorineural** (central disease in inner ear, cochlea, or nerve)
- Ototoxic deafness caused by streptomycin, neomycin, and quinine

CN IX (Glossopharyngeal)

- Primarily sensory (oropharynx/palate, middle ear, taste from posterior one-third of tongue)
- Autonomic input from **carotid sinus** (baroreceptors for blood pressure) and **carotid body** (chemoreceptors for blood CO_2 and O_2 concentration)
- Innervates pharyngeal muscle used in swallowing (**stylopharyngeus**)
- **Afferent limb of gag reflex**
- Provides parasympathetic innervation from **salivatory nucleus** to parotid gland
- Visceral sensory input goes to **nucleus solitarius**
- Derived from brachial arch 3
- Exits skull with CN X and XI through **jugular foramen**

CN X (Vagus)

- Autonomic: **Parasympathetic** input to smooth muscles of the heart, blood vessels, trachea, bronchi, esophagus, stomach, and intestine
- Motor input to pharyngeal arch muscles of larynx and pharynx, striated muscle of upper esophagus, uvula (**efferent limb of gag reflex**); visceral input to organs of neck, thoracic, and abdominal cavities; somatic input to muscles of larynx via cranial division of CN XI
- Receives somatic input from infratentorial dura, external ear, external auditory meatus, and tympanic membrane; projects central processes to spinal trigeminal tract
- Receives visceral input from pharynx, larynx, esophagus, trachea, thoracic, and abdominal viscera to the left of colic flexure
- Sensory input from taste buds on epiglottis
- Derived from brachial arches 4 and 6
- Exits skull via **jugular foramen**

CN XI (Accessory)

- Input to **trapezius** and **sternocleidomastoid** muscles
- Innervates muscles of larynx through CN X
- Exits skull via **jugular foramen**

CN XII (Hypoglossal)

- Innervates **intrinsic and extrinsic muscles of tongue**
- Passes through hypoglossal canal
- Transection of lower motor nerve results in **tongue deviation toward the side of the lesion**, due to unopposed action of contralateral genioglossus muscle
- Upper motor neuron lesion results in deviation of tongue **away** from side of lesion

Cranial Nerve Functions

- *Cranial nerves can have just one or many different functions*

Efferent (Motor)

- Sending message *from CNS to periphery* (*"e" for "exit"* the CNS)
  - ○ General somatic efferent (GSE): Skeletal muscle/somites
  - ○ General visceral efferent (GVE): Autonomic control
  - ○ Special visceral efferent (SVE): Branchiomeric skeletal muscles

Afferent (Sensory)

- Bringing information *from periphery to CNS*
  - ○ General somatic afferent (GSA): Touch, pain, temperature, proprioception
  - ○ General visceral afferent (GVA): Pain, temperature, and proprioception from internal structures
  - ○ Special somatic afferent (SSA): Vision, hearing, equilibrium
  - ○ Special visceral afferent (SVA): Smell, taste

  Mnemonic (in order of cranial nerves I to XII):

  Some Say Money Matters But My Brother Says Big Brains Matter Most
  (S = sensory, M = motor, B = both)

TABLE 6-1 Functional Constituents of the Cranial Nerves

CRANIAL NERVE	GSE	GVE (ALL PARASYMPATHETIC)	SVE	GSA	GVA	SSA	SVA
Sensory (Afferent)							
I							●
II						●	
VIII						●	
Motor (Efferent)							
III	●	●					
IV	●						
VI	●						
XI	●						
XII	●						
Both Sensory and Motor							
V			●	●	●		
VII		●	●	●	●		●
IX		●	●	●	●		●
X		●	●	●	●		●

CHAPTER 7

Spinal Cord and Peripheral Nerves

The spinal cord is the main pathway connecting the brain and peripheral nervous system. Its anatomy allows for coordinated sensation and movement, with spinal cord circuits serving to integrate ascending and descending information. Damage to structures of the cord results in well-described clinical syndromes.

GROSS ANATOMY

The spinal cord is located inside the vertebral canal, surrounded by the foramina of:

- 7 cervical vertebrae
- 12 thoracic vertebrae
- 5 lumbar vertebrae
- 5 sacral vertebrae

Mnemonic: Breakfast at 7, lunch at 12, dinner (twice!) at 5

The cord itself is composed of 31 segments:

- 8 cervical (C)
- 12 thoracic (T)
- 5 lumbar (L)
- 5 sacral (S)
- 1 coccygeal
- Ends at level of *L1 and L2* vertebrae
- *Conus medullaris* is cone-shaped termination of spinal cord
- *Cauda equina* (Latin for horse tail) is collection of lumbar and sacral spinal nerve roots below the conus medullaris
  - Roots travel caudally in the subarachnoid space
- Pia mater continues caudally as *filum terminale*
- Cord is "fatter" in the cervical and lumbosacral segments as a result of upper and lower limb innervation
- Cell bodies of *motor neurons* are located in the *anterior horn* within the cord parenchyma
- Cell bodies of *sensory neurons* are found in the *dorsal root ganglia*
- *Sensory nerve roots* (dorsal roots) enter the spinal cord *dorsally* at each level
- *Motor roots* (ventral roots) emerge *ventrally* from the cord at each level

HARDCORE

Cauda equina syndrome develops from compression of the cauda equina, which can occur with *tumors* or *lumbar disk prolapse*, results in *flaccid weakness*, *sensory loss* (*saddle anesthesia*), *areflexia*, and possible *bowel/bladder symptoms*. One or both sides may be affected, depending on whether compression is midline or not. Bladder symptoms may include *overflow incontinence*, resulting from *loss of parasympathetic innervation* to bladder.

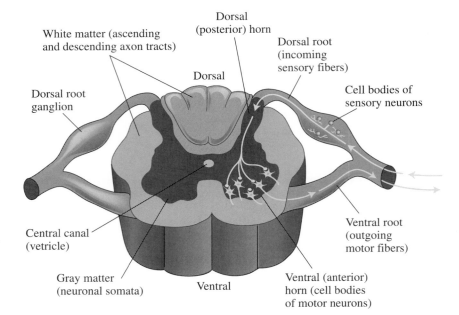

Figure 7-1 The anatomical organization of the spinal cord. Sensory roots emerge from the dorsal root ganglion and enter the cord dorsally, while motor roots exit the cord ventrally. (Reprinted with permission from Matthews GG. Neurobiology: Molecules, Cells, Systems. 2nd ed. Malden, MA: Blackwell Publishing, 2001:167.)

HARDCORE

- Nerves from C1 to C7 emerge above their respective vertebrae
- C8 emerges between the seventh cervical and first thoracic vertebrae
- T1 and below exit beneath their respective vertebrae

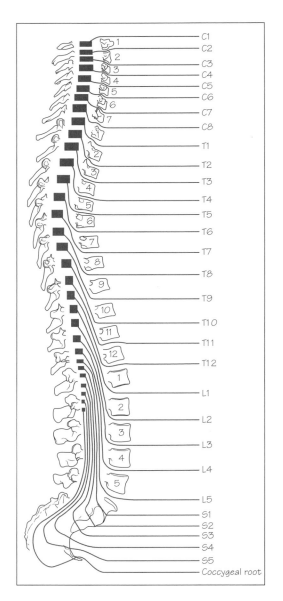

Figure 7-2 Anatomical relationship between vertebrae and spinal nerves. (Reprinted with permission from Ginsberg L. Lecture Notes: Neurology. 8th ed. Oxford: Blackwell Publishing, 2005:126.)

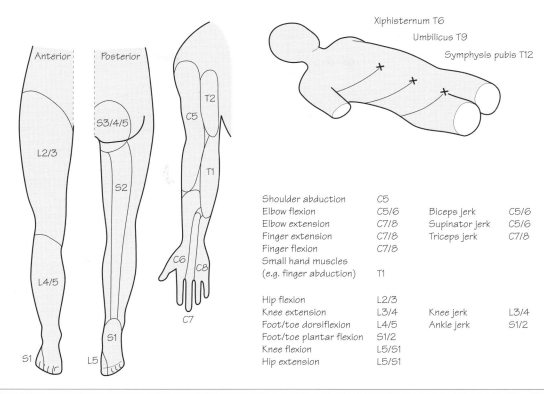

Figure 7-3 Clinically important dermatomes, maps that portray sensory distributions from each level. (Reprinted with permission from Wilkinson I. Essential Neurology. 4th ed. Oxford: Blackwell Publishing, 2005:89.)

Vascular Supply to the Spinal Cord

- Originates superiorly from the **vertebral arteries** and, in the low cervical and thoracic area, from **branches of the aorta**
- The anterior spinal artery supplies the **anterior two-thirds** of the cord
- The posterior spinal artery supplies the **posterior one-third** of the cord
- Radicular arteries supply roots

IMPORTANT TRACTS OF THE SPINAL CORD

- **External** portion of the spinal cord consists of **white matter** (myelinated nerves)
  - Contains ascending and descending tracts of longitudinally oriented axons
  - Tracts are named by a composite of their origin and destination
- **Internal** portion consists of **gray matter**
  - Divided into **anterior/ventral horn (motor)**, **posterior/dorsal horn (sensory)**, and **lateral horn neurons (found from T1–L2 only; sympathetic motor)**

Main Tracts

Pyramidal

- Also known as the **corticospinal tract (CST)**
- Descending fibers from layer V of cerebral cortex (**motor homunculus**) cross in **lower medulla** (at pyramidal decussation) and innervate lower motor neurons in the **contralateral ventral horn**

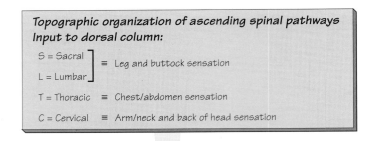

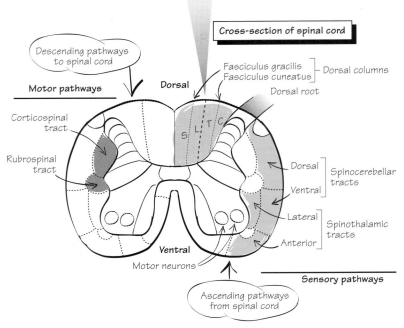

Figure 7-4 Important tracts of the spinal cord.
(Modified with permission from Barker RA. Neuroscience at a Glance. 2nd ed. Oxford: Blackwell Publishing, 2003:32.)

HARDCORE

Pyramidal:

- Transection above the decussation results in contralateral spastic paresis and Babinski's sign
- Transection in the spinal cord results in ipsilateral spastic paresis and Babinski's sign (upgoing toes)

HARDCORE

Dorsal column:

- Transection above the decussation results in contralateral loss of sensory modalities below the lesion
- Transection in the spinal cord results in ipsilateral loss

HARDCORE

Lateral spinothalamic:

- Transection results in contralateral loss of pain and temperature below the lesion

Dorsal Column

- Ascending fibers carrying *proprioception* and *vibration* sense from the *lower (gracile fasciculus)* and *upper (cuneate fasciculus) extremities*
- Fibers cross to *contralateral* side in the medulla
- Terminates in *ventral posterolateral nucleus of thalamus* and sensory cortex

Lateral Spinothalamic

- Ascending fibers from dorsal horn neurons carry *pain and temperature* sense
- Cross in the *ventral white commissure* (of spinal cord) to reach *contralateral* thalamus and sensory cortex

SPINAL REFLEXES

- A simple, stereotyped motor response to a defined sensory input
- Circuit occurs in spinal cord without involvement of brain
- Stretch reflex responds to passive stretching of muscle
  - Has an afferent (muscle spindle/receptor, dorsal root ganglion, and its Ia fibers) and an efferent (ventral horn motor neurons and the muscles they innervate) limb
  - Interruption of either limb results in areflexia
  - Important for maintenance of posture and muscle tone, but higher control through upper motor neurons can influence the reflex

TABLE 7-1	Commonly Tested Muscle Stretch Reflexes	
REFLEX	SPINAL CORD SEGMENT	CORRESPONDING MUSCLE
Knee	L2–L4	Quadriceps
Ankle	S1	Gastrocnemius
Biceps, forearm	C5 and C6	Biceps, brachioradialis
Triceps	C7 and C8	Triceps

Know the commonly tested muscle stretch reflexes listed in Table 7.1

UPPER AND LOWER MOTOR NEURON SYNDROMES

Upper Motor Neuron (UMN) Lesions

Caused by transection of the CST or damage to neurons in the cerebral cortex. Characteristics include:

- Spasticity
- Increased tone
- Weakness (especially in antigravity muscles)
- *Hyperreflexia* and clonus
- *Extensor plantar responses (Babinski's sign)*
- *No associated muscle atrophy or wasting*

Lower Motor Neuron (LMN) Lesions

Reflect damage at the level of the spinal ventral neurons. Characteristics include:

- Either the cell body and/or the axon may be involved
- *Muscle atrophy (wasting)*
- Muscle fasciculation
- Decreased tone (*flaccidity*)
- Weakness
- *Hyporeflexia* or absent reflexes
- *Flexor (downgoing toes)* or *absent plantar responses*

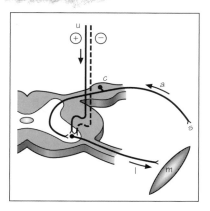

Figure 7-5 Schematic of a reflex arc. (Reprinted with permission from Ginsberg L. Lecture Notes: Neurology. 8th ed. Oxford: Blackwell Publishing, 2005:39.)

TABLE 7-2	Summary Comparison of UMN and LMN Lesions	
	UMN LESION	LMN LESION
Atrophy	No	Yes
Tendon reflexes	Hyperreflexia	Decreased or absent
Fasiculations	No	Yes
Clonus	Yes	No
Muscle tone	Increased	Decreased
Plantar response	Upgoing	Downgoing
Posture	Drift of outstretched arm with eyes closed (pronator drift)	N/A

CLASSIC SPINAL CORD SYNDROMES

In most instances, incomplete forms are far more common.

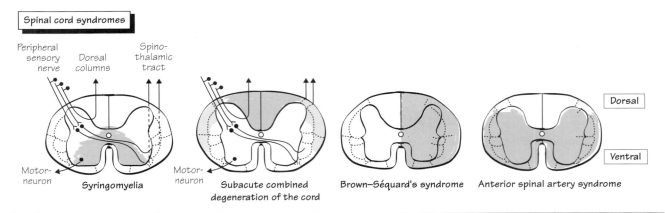

Figure 7-6 Spinal cord syndromes. (Modified with permission from Barker RA. Neuroscience at a Glance. 2nd ed. Oxford: Blackwell Publishing, 2003:70.)

Syringomyelia

- Development of *cyst or cavity near central canal*, usually in *cervical region* of spinal cord
- Results in *dissociated sensory loss* (loss of pain/temperature sense with intact proprioception/vibration sense) due to *disruption of spinothalamic tract fibers as they cross spinal cord ventral to the central canal*
- Expansion of cyst/cavity into ventral horn can result in motor involvement

Subacute Combined Degeneration of the Spinal Cord

- Usually associated with *pernicious anemia* or *vitamin B$_{12}$ deficiency*
- Characterized by *demyelination/degeneration of dorsal columns, corticospinal tract, spinocerebellar tracts, and peripheral nerves*
- Results in combination of *paresthesias and sensory loss* with *weakness and incoordination*

Brown-Séquard's Syndrome

- Results from hemicordectomy, usually secondary to trauma
- Ipsilateral spastic paresis and flaccid muscular paralysis
- Ipsilateral loss of vibration and position sense below level of lesion
- Contralateral loss of pain and temperature below level of lesion
- Ipsilateral hyperreflexia and Babinski's sign

Anterior Spinal Artery Syndrome

- Typically due to anterior spinal artery infarction
- Results in bilateral paralysis and bilateral loss of pain and temperature below level of lesion
- Relative sparing of touch, vibration, and position sense (because dorsal columns receive their primary blood supply from the posterior spinal arteries)

Radiculopathy Syndromes

- Caused by damage to nerve root
- Dorsal root involvement results in dermatomal sensory changes
- Ventral root involvement results in myotomal weakness
- Radicular pain (shooting pain) usually increases with increased intraspinal pressure (coughing, sneezing, any Valsalva maneuver)

PERIPHERAL NERVE DISORDERS

Mononeuropathies

- Damage to individual peripheral nerve, typically secondary to trauma, pressure, or damaged blood supply

HARDCORE

Tabes dorsalis is a lesion of sensory pathways seen in **neurosyphilis**.

- Demyelination of dorsal roots results in loss of tactile discrimination and position and vibration sense, as well as pain and paresthesias
- **Positive Romberg's sign** (dorsal column ataxia)

Carpal Tunnel Syndrome

- Compression of *median nerve* at wrist as it passes through carpal tunnel
- Occurs in patients with manual occupations
- Clinical features: Pain in hand/arm; *wasting/weakness of thenar eminence muscles*; sensory loss in distribution of median nerve; tingling paresthesias following percussion of carpal tunnel (Tinel's sign)
- Treatment: Splinting, steroids, surgical decompression

Ulnar Neuropathy

- Ulnar nerve is particularly sensitive to damage at elbow
- Clinical features: Pain/tingling radiating from elbow down forearm; wasting/weakness of intrinsic hand muscles (*sparing thenar eminence*)
- Characteristic "*claw-hand deformity*"

Radial Palsy

- Results from pressure on *radial nerve* (e.g., from resting arm over chair while intoxicated, the so-called "*Saturday night palsy*")
- May lead to *acute wrist drop*

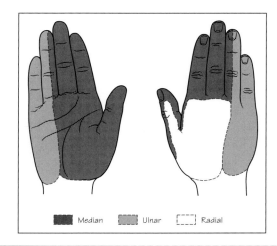

Median | Ulnar | Radial

Figure 7-7 Sensory loss in the hand (cutaneous distributions of median, ulnar, and radial nerve). (Reprinted with permission from Ginsberg L. Lecture Notes: Neurology. 8th ed. Oxford: Blackwell Publishing, 2005:138.)

HARDCORE

Upper plexus lesion (Erb's palsy):

- Typically results from birth injury or trauma (e.g., motorcycle accident)
- C5–C6 dysfunction causes palsy of deltoids, biceps, supraspinatus and infraspinatus, with difficulty abducting shoulder and flexing elbow, and C5–C6 sensory loss

HARDCORE

Lower plexus lesion (Klumpke's palsy)

- C8–T1 damage leads to intrinsic hand muscle weakness and C8–T1 sensory loss

HARDCORE

Thoracic outlet syndrome

- Results from compression of *brachial plexus, subclavian artery and vein*, possibly from anomalous structures like cervical rib or congenital fibrous band
- Presents with neck/shoulder pain, forearm paresthesias, intrinsic hand muscle weakness

HARDCORE

Long thoracic nerve palsy

- Damage to C5, C6, and C7 results in *serratus anterior* palsy, leading to *winging of the scapula* (may be seen postoperatively, e.g., after axillary node dissection)

HARDCORE

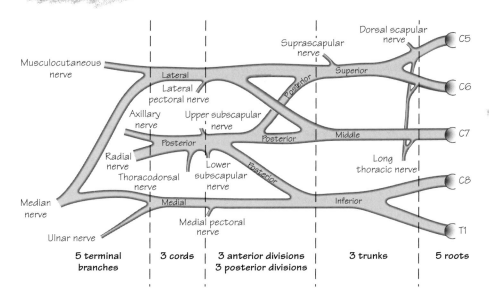

Figure 7-8 Brachial plexus (*Note: Smaller nerve branches have been omitted for simplicity*). (Reprinted with permission from Wechsler RT. Blueprints Notes & Cases: Neuroscience. Malden, MA: Blackwell Publishing, 2004:152.)

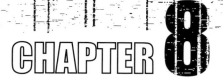

CHAPTER 8

Autonomic Nervous System

The "autonomic nervous system" (ANS) is so named because of its seemingly "autonomous" function, the ANS regulates the internal body milieu by exerting control over cardiac and smooth muscle, glandular function, blood flow, and digestion.

ORGANIZATION OF THE AUTONOMIC NERVOUS SYSTEM

- Divided into *sympathetic* and *parasympathetic* divisions
- Divisions differ in terms of anatomy, neurotransmitters employed, and physiological effects

Sympathetic System

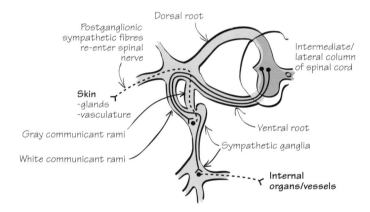

Figure 8-1 **The sympathetic fibers leaving the lateral columns in the spinal cord via the anterior (ventral) nerve root.** The fibers form the white rami communicantes and either continue to synapse in ganglia of the sympathetic trunk, or synapse and return to join spinal nerves through the gray rami communicantes. (Reprinted with permission from Barker RA. Neuroscience at a Glance. 2nd ed. Blackwell Publishing, 2003:92.)

Anatomy

EFFERENT FIBERS

- *Efferent* fibers (or thoracolumbar outflow) originate in the *lateral gray columns* (horns) of the spinal cord *between T1 and L2–L3*
  - Myelinated axons leave the cord via the anterior (ventral) nerve root (forming the *white rami communicantes*)
- Most of these preganglionic fibers synapse in the *paravertebral ganglia* of the sympathetic trunk (a ganglionated nerve trunk that travels the entire length on both sides of the spinal cord)
- Postganglionic nonmyelinated fibers (forming the *gray rami communicantes*) leave the ganglion and travel to thoracic spinal nerves
- These fibers travel with branches of the thoracic spinal nerves to reach smooth muscle in blood vessel walls, sweat glands, and erector muscle of hairs
- Some preganglionic fibers *travel up or down in the sympathetic trunk* before synapsing, allowing for sympathetic fibers to reach cervical and sacral regions
- Other preganglionic fibers do not synapse in the sympathetic trunk, but leave and synapse in various plexuses; e.g., some myelinated fibers leave the trunk as the *greater splanchnic nerve* and synapse in the ganglia of the *celiac plexus*, the *renal plexus*, and the suprarenal medulla

AFFERENT FIBERS

- *Afferent* fibers travel from the viscera through the sympathetic ganglia
  - ○ Myelinated fibers pass through the white rami communicantes and reach their cell bodies in the *dorsal root ganglion* of the corresponding spinal nerve
  - ○ Central axons can enter spinal cord or ascend to higher centers such as the hypothalamus

Neurotransmitters

- *Preganglionic* neurons use *acetylcholine* to activate postganglionic neurons (which have either nicotinic or muscarinic receptors)
- Most *postganglionic* neurons use *norepinephrine* to exert their effect on effector organs, although some (e.g., those that innervate sweat glands and blood vessels in skeletal muscle) use acetylcholine
- Sympathetic nerves that utilize norepinephrine are termed *adrenergic*; the released norepinephrine interacts with either *α or β receptors on effector organs*
  - ○ α receptors include types 1 and 2
  - ○ β receptors include types 1 and 2
  - ○ Neurotransmitters activate these receptors to different degrees
    - Phenylephrine: Pure α stimulator
    - Albuterol: Mainly β2 stimulator

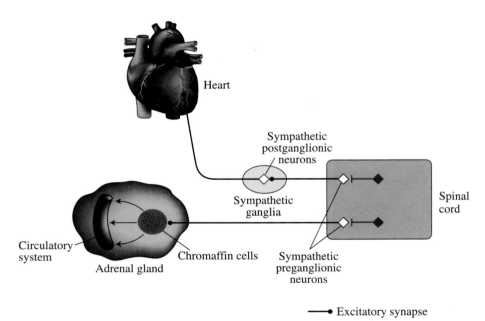

Figure 8-2 An adrenergic sympathetic neuron.
The preganglionic neuron releases acetylcholine, which interacts with nicotinic receptors on the postganglionic neuron. The postganglionic neuron releases epinephrine, which stimulates either α or β receptors on effector organs. Preganglionic sympathetic neurons stimulate the adrenal gland directly without synapsing in a ganglion first. (Modified with permission from Matthews GG. Neurobiology: Molecules, Cells, Systems. 2nd ed. Malden, MA: Blackwell Publishing, 2001:255.)

Functions

- In general, the sympathetic nervous system is responsible for the "fight or flight" response
- Dilation of pupils (α1 receptors)
- Increase in heart rate, force of contraction, and blood pressure (β1 and β2 receptors)
- Arterioles to skin/intestine constrict (α receptors)
- Increased blood flow to skeletal and cardiac muscle (β2 receptors)
- Airways dilate (β2 receptors)
- Blood glucose level increases via gluconeogenesis and glycogenolysis in liver (β2 and α receptors)

Parasympathetic System

Anatomy

- *Efferent fibers* (or craniosacral outflow) originate from the brainstem and sacral segments of the spinal cord (recall the term *"para"*; the parasympathetic system is literally para to the sympathetic system in terms of anatomical origin)

HARDCORE

Any *disruption along the pathway of sympathetic innervation* to the face results in the classic triad of *ptosis, miosis, and anhydrosis* (Horner's syndrome). One cause is a *Pancoast tumor* (involving the apex of the lung), which can compress the *superior cervical ganglion*.

- *Parasympathetic nerve cells form nuclei in some of the cranial nerves* (CNs), and their axons travel within the cranial nerves themselves:
  - Oculomotor (CN III): Parasympathetic or Edinger-Westphal nucleus
  - Facial (CN VII): Superior salivatory nucleus and lacrimatory nucleus
  - Glossopharyngeal (CN IX): Inferior salivatory nucleus
  - Vagus (CN X): Dorsal nucleus of the vagus
- *Sacral nerve cells are found in gray matter of S2–S4*
  - Myelinated axons leave cord in anterior nerve roots of corresponding spinal nerves
- Myelinated efferent fibers synapse in *peripheral ganglia close to the viscera they innervate*
  - Some of these peripheral ganglia are organized into *plexuses*
- *Afferent* parasympathetic fibers travel from the viscera to their cell bodies, in either the *sensory ganglia of cranial nerves* or the *dorsal root ganglia of the sacrospinal nerves*

Neurotransmitters

- Preganglionic *and* postganglionic neurons utilize *acetylcholine* as a neurotransmitter

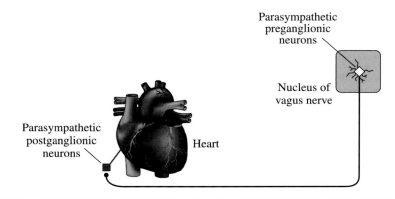

Figure 8-3 Cholinergic neuron. All parasympathetic neurons release acetylcholine at both the pre- and postsynaptic nerve terminals. (Modified with permission from Matthews GG. Neurobiology: Molecules, Cells, Systems. 2nd ed. Malden, MA: Blackwell Publishing, 2001:255.)

Functions

- The parasympathetic system is responsible for "resting and digesting"
- *SLUDD:*
  - Salivation
  - Lacrimation
  - Urination
  - Digestion
  - Defecation
  - Also decreases heart rate, diameter of airways and pupils

HARDCORE

Most viscera receive innervation from autonomic nerves instead of somatic nerves. Pain conducted along these autonomic nerves is often diffuse and poorly localized, making visceral pain "dull" in contrast to "sharp" somatic pain. Often, such *pain is felt at skin areas that are innervated by the same segments of the spinal cord as the painful viscus*. For example, visceral pain impulses from the gallbladder travel with sympathetic fibers through the celiac plexus to segments T5–T9 of the spinal cord. The pain is often referred to the lower chest and upper abdomen—the dermatomal areas supplied by those spinal cord segments (T5–T9). Similarly, cardiac pain is carried by nerve fibers through the cardiac plexus and sympathetic chain to dorsal root ganglia of T1–T4. These spinal cord segments supply cutaneous innervation to neck, jaw, shoulder, arms, and stomach, commonly resulting in pain perception in these areas during myocardial infarction.

RECEPTORS AND PHARMACOLOGY OF THE ANS

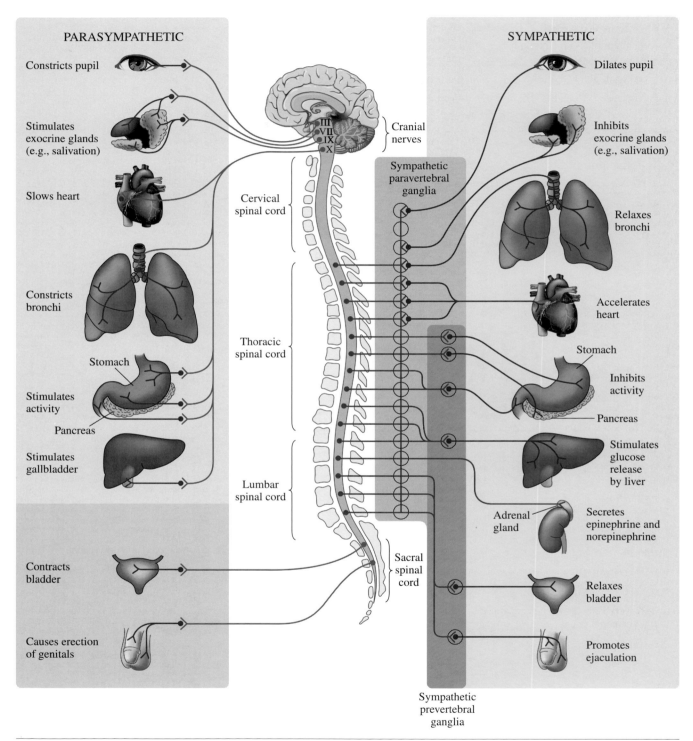

PARASYMPATHETIC

Constricts pupil

Stimulates exocrine glands (e.g., salivation)

Slows heart

Constricts bronchi

Stomach

Stimulates activity

Pancreas

Stimulates gallbladder

Contracts bladder

Causes erection of genitals

Cranial nerves

Cervical spinal cord

Thoracic spinal cord

Lumbar spinal cord

Sacral spinal cord

Sympathetic paravertebral ganglia

Sympathetic prevertebral ganglia

SYMPATHETIC

Dilates pupil

Inhibits exocrine glands (e.g., salivation)

Relaxes bronchi

Accelerates heart

Stomach

Inhibits activity

Pancreas

Stimulates glucose release by liver

Adrenal gland

Secretes epinephrine and norepinephrine

Relaxes bladder

Promotes ejaculation

Figure 8-4 Organization of ANS. Note that the sympathetic trunk contains ganglia that travel along the spinal cord. Shorter preganglionic fibers exit the white rami communicantes and synapse here, while the postganglionic fibers circle back to the spinal cord through the gray rami communicantes and travel with the spinal nerves. Some preganglionic fibers do not synapse until reaching a plexus distal to the sympathetic trunk. In contrast to the sympathetic system, the parasympathetic nerves originate from the "top" and "bottom" of the spinal cord, and preganglionic fibers travel to the site of action, where they synapse with ganglia near the effector organ. (Modified with permission from Matthews GG. Neurobiology: Molecules, Cells, Systems. 2nd ed. Malden, MA: Blackwell Publishing, 2001:252.)

TABLE 8-1	Receptors and Effector Organs in the ANS					
ORGAN	PARASYMPATHETIC			SYMPATHETIC		
	Action	Innervation	Receptor	Action	Innervation	Receptor
Eye	Pupillary constriction (miosis)	CN III via ciliary ganglion	M3 (muscarinic)	Pupillary dilation (mydriasis)	T1–T2 via superior cervical ganglion	α1
Heart	• Decreased contractility • Decreased rate	CN X	M2	• Increased contractility • Increased rate	T1–T6	β1, β2
Bronchial tree	Bronchoconstriction and increased secretion	CN X	M3	Bronchodilation and decreased secretion	T3–T6	β2
Skin and splanchnic vessels				Contraction		α
Skeletal muscle vessels				Relaxation		β2
Adrenal gland				Preganglionic fibers synapse directly on gland, causing catecholamine release	T8–T11	
Lower bowel	Contraction	S2–S4 sacral plexus	M3	Inhibition of peristalsis	T9–L2	β2
NEUROTRANSMITTERS						
Preganglionic	Acetylcholine			Acetylcholine		
Postganglionic	Acetylcholine			Norepinephrine		

Cholinergic Receptors

- Respond to *acetylcholine*
- Two types of cholinergic receptors are *muscarinic* and *nicotinic*
  - Most muscarinic receptors are innervated by *parasympathetic nerves* and are found throughout the body
  - Nicotinic receptors are found at ganglia and *neuromuscular junctions*

Cholinomimetics

- Agents that act like acetylcholine

DIRECT ACETYLCHOLINE AGONISTS

- Esters of choline and alkaloids
  - Bethanechol
  - Pilocarpine

INDIRECT ACETYLCHOLINESTERASE INHIBITORS

- Edrophonium: Short-acting, used in diagnosis of myasthenia gravis (Tensilon test)
- Neostigmine
- Organophosphates (including pesticides parathion and malathion)

Anticholinergics

ANTIMUSCARINICS

- *Atropine* (called "belladonna"; was used in past to dilate women's pupils for cosmetic effect)
  - Salivary, bronchial, and sweat glands most sensitive
  - Used in past as treatment for Parkinson's disease to balance out relative excess of cholinergic activity

ANTINICOTINICS

- Tubocurarine (neuromuscular end-plate blocker)
- Hexamethonium (ganglion blocker)

HARDCORE

Overdosing on cholinomimetics, such as organophosphate pesticides, leads to characteristic symptoms: *DUMBELSS*

- **D**iarrhea
- **U**rination
- **M**iosis
- **B**ronchospasm
- **E**xcitation
- **L**acrimation
- **S**weating
- **S**alivation

Treatment: Atropine (see discussion of antimuscarinics) or pralidoxime.

HARDCORE

Atropine toxicity: *Dry as a bone, blind as a bat, red as a beet, mad as a hatter.*

Adrenergic Receptors

- Respond to *norepinephrine*
- Four main adrenoreceptors: $\alpha 1$, $\alpha 2$, $\beta 1$, $\beta 2$

Sympathomimetics

- Activate adrenoreceptors
- Agents have different affinities for specific receptors:
  - *Epinephrine* acts on $\alpha 1$, $\alpha 2$, $\beta 1$, and $\beta 2$
  - *Norepinephrine* acts on α and $\beta 1$
  - *Phenylephrine* acts on $\alpha 1$ and $\alpha 2$
  - *Isoproterenol* acts on β
  - *Dopamine* acts on dopamine receptors $> \beta > \alpha$
- β agonists cause increased heart rate but can result in a drop in blood pressure because of vasodilation of skeletal muscle vessels
- β agonist plus an α agonist, however, increase blood pressure because of constriction of vessels mediated through α receptors (as seen with pharmacologic doses of epinephrine, where α effects predominate over β effects)

Sympathoplegics

- α-Blockers
  - Phenoxybenzamine
  - Prazosin ($\alpha 1$ blocker; used in benign prostatic hypertrophy)
- β-Blockers
- Some are selective for $\beta 1$, while others inhibit both $\beta 1$ and $\beta 2$
- Examples of $\beta 1$-selective drugs:
  - Atenolol, esmolol, metoprolol
- Examples of nonselective drugs:
  - Labetalol, propanolol, timolol

ENTERIC NERVOUS SYSTEM

The enteric nervous system is often considered a third branch of the autonomic nervous system.

- Composed of *two plexuses* of nerve cells and fibers extending continuously along the length of the gastrointestinal tract
- *Parasympathetic innervation* carried by vagus and pelvic nerves, although coordinated contractions can occur in isolation from central nervous system
- *Sympathetic preganglionic fibers* synapse in several splanchnic ganglia (passing through sympathetic trunk without synapsing)
  - *Submucosal plexus (Meissner's plexus)*
    - Located between mucosa and inner circular muscle layer
  - *Myenteric plexus (Auerbach's plexus)*
    - Located between inner circular muscle and outer longitudinal muscle layers
  - Functions:
    - **S**ubmucosal plexus involved in **S**ecretions
    - **M**yenteric plexus involved in **M**otility

AUTONOMIC CONTROL

The *hypothalamus* influences the ANS and integrates autonomic and neuroendocrine systems.

- Stimulation of *anterior* hypothalamic area induces *parasympathetic* responses
- Stimulation of *posterior and lateral* nuclei induces *sympathetic* responses
- Other hypothalamic functions:
  - Release of *regulatory hormones* that act on the pituitary
  - Synthesis of *antidiuretic hormone and oxytocin*
  - Control of temperature, hunger, satiety, thirst, and circadian rhythms

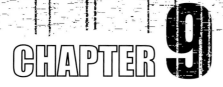

Sensory Systems

Sensory information arising from the skin, muscles, and joints travels through the nervous system in specific tracts along the spinal cord. These ascending tracts allow for integration of sensory information by the central nervous system and function to allow for proper responses to various stimuli.

SENSORY RECEPTORS

- Sensation begins at somatic and visceral nerve endings (**peripheral nociceptors**)
- Different types of receptors/nerve endings transmit different sensations
  - **Nociceptors**: Free nerve endings that detect pain
  - **Merkel's discs**: Detect touch and pressure
  - **Meissner's corpuscles**: Two-point tactile discrimination
  - **Pacinian corpuscles**: "Onion skin" shaped receptors that detect pressure and vibration
  - **Neuromuscular spindles**: Detect elongation of muscle (stretch)

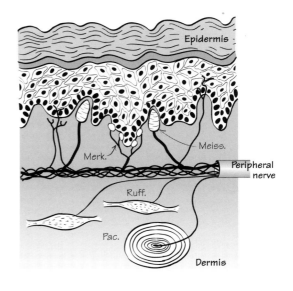

Classification of cutaneous receptors		
	Speed of adaptation of receptor	
Size of receptive field	Rapid (RA)	Slow (SA)
Type I Small, sharp, well defined receptive fields —mainly found on fingertips	RA^I Meissner's corpuscle (Meiss.)	SA^I Merkel's disc (Merk.)
Type II Large, poorly defined receptive fields	RA^{II} Pacinian corpuscle (Pac.)	SA^{II} Ruffini ending (Ruff.)

Figure 9-1 **Distribution of cutaneous receptors in hairless skin.** (Modified with permission from Barker RA. Neuroscience at a Glance. 2nd ed. Oxford: Blackwell Publishing, 2003:48.)

ASCENDING TRACTS OF THE SPINAL CORD

Lateral Spinothalamic Tract

- **Carries pain and temperature impulses via fast delta A-type fibers and slow C-type fibers**
- Fibers of dorsal root **enter cord anterolaterally** and ascend a few segments in **Lissauer's tract**
- After synapsing in dorsal horn, **fibers cross to opposite side** and ascend in contralateral white column as lateral spinothalamic tract
- Travels to **thalamus**, where fibers synapse, and impulses are carried further to cerebral cortex
- Neurotransmitters that activate peripheral nociceptors: Substance P, bradykinins, prostaglandins, histamine

HARDCORE

- Typically, sensory input **begins at sensory receptor** and travels via first-order neuron to synapse in **dorsal root ganglion** of spinal nerve
- Second-order neuron **decussates** (crosses to opposite side of spinal cord) and ascends, often synapsing in **thalamus**
- Third-order neuron in thalamus projects to **sensory** region of cerebral cortex

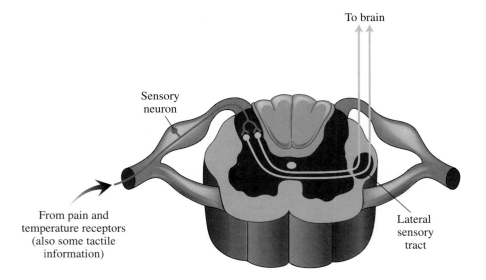

Sensory neuron

To brain

From pain and temperature receptors (also some tactile information)

Lateral sensory tract

Figure 9-2 Schematic diagram showing projection pattern of sensory information in lateral spinothalamic tract. (Reprinted with permission from Matthews GG. Neurobiology: Molecules, Cells, Systems. 2nd ed. Malden, MA: Blackwell Publishing, 2001:304.)

Anterior Spinothalamic Tract

- *Carries light touch and pressure*
- Axons enter spinal cord from dorsal root ganglion and travel in *Lissauer's tract*
- Fibers synapse in *posterior gray column* and cross to opposite side
- Fibers ascend as anterior spinothalamic tract
- Forms *spinal lemniscus* with lateral spinothalamic tract and spinotectal tract
- Fibers synapse in *ventral posterolateral nucleus of thalamus*
- Third-order neurons pass through internal capsule and corona radiate, carrying crude touch/pressure awareness to cerebral cortex

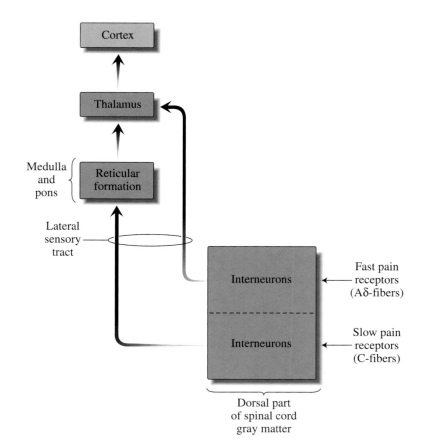

Cortex

Thalamus

Medulla and pons

Reticular formation

Lateral sensory tract

Interneurons

Fast pain receptors (Aδ-fibers)

Interneurons

Slow pain receptors (C-fibers)

Dorsal part of spinal cord gray matter

Figure 9-3 Organization of the anterolateral system. Note that impulses carried by slow C-type fibers connect diffusely to reticular formation of brainstem, while fast delta A-type fibers project directly to thalamus. (Reprinted with permission from Matthews GG. Neurobiology: Molecules, Cells, Systems. 2nd ed. Malden, MA: Blackwell Publishing, 2001:307.)

Dorsal Columns

FASCICULUS GRACILIS AND FASCICULUS CUNEATUS

- *Carry discriminative touch, vibratory sense, and proprioception (conscious muscle/joint position)*
- Muscle spindles, joint, and cutaneous receptors transmit sensory information to dorsal root ganglion
- Input from sacral, lumbar, and lower thoracic spinal nerves travels as fasciculus gracilis
- Input from upper thoracic and cervical segments travels as fasciculus cuneatus (lateral to fasciculus gracilis—think that arms are "lateral" to the legs)
- Impulses travel *without* crossing (ipsilaterally) and synapse in medulla at nucleus gracilis and nucleus cuneatus, respectively
- Now, second-order neurons *decussate*, passing through the medial lemniscus and synapsing in thalamus
- Impulse passes through internal capsule on way to cortex

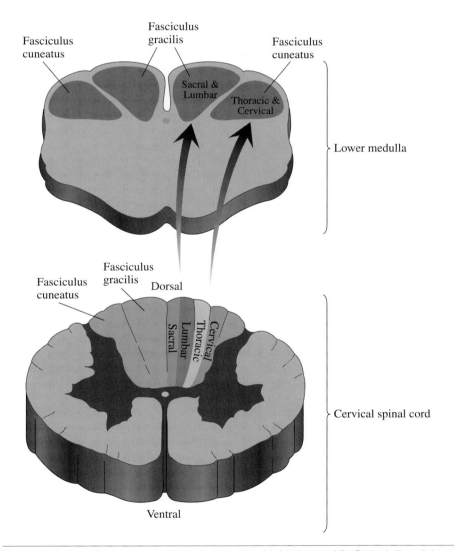

Figure 9-4 Projections of the dorsal columns into the dorsal column nuclei of the lower medulla. (Reprinted with permission from Matthews GG. Neurobiology: Molecules, Cells, Systems. 2nd ed. Malden, MA: Blackwell Publishing, 2001:306.)

Spinocerebellar Tract

- *Carries proprioception from trunk and lower limbs (muscle stretch, joint position)*
- Fibers from dorsal root ganglion enter cord and travel in dorsal horn
- Fibers synapse in *Clark's column* (nucleus dorsalis)
- Some secondary afferents that travel in *dorsal spinocerebellar tract* stay ipsilateral and join fibers from inferior olive, forming *inferior cerebellar peduncle*
- Other secondary afferents travel in *ventral spinocerebellar tract*, cross the midline at level of dorsal root, and cross back again in pons, forming *superior cerebellar peduncle*
- Fibers *terminate in cerebellar cortex*

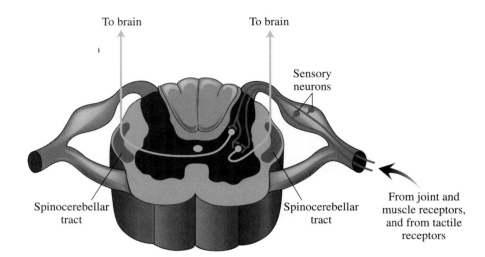

Figure 9-5 Projection pattern of sensory information in spinocerebellar tracts. (Reprinted with permission from Matthews GG. Neurobiology: Molecules, Cells, Systems. 2nd ed. Malden, MA: Blackwell Publishing, 2001:304.)

Other Sensory Pathways

TRIGEMINAL SYSTEM (CN V)

- Contains both sensory and motor fibers
- Sensory nucleus: Long structure that extends into medulla and receives information from three branches on face
  - **Ophthalmic**
  - **Maxillary**
  - **Mandibular**
- Impulses of pain, temperature, touch, and pressure enter and synapse on *ipsilateral pons*
- Fibers then cross to *contralateral trigeminal lemniscus and synapse at thalamus*

VESTIBULAR NUCLEAR COMPLEX

- Group of four nuclei beneath the fourth ventricle
  - Lateral, superior, medial, and inferior vestibular nuclei
  - Receive afferent fibers from *utricle, saccule, and semicircular canals*
  - Input comes from vestibular nerve and cerebellar fibers via inferior cerebellar peduncle
  - These connections allow for *coordination of head and eye movement, necessary for visual fixation, and balance*

COCHLEAR NUCLEI

- Cochlear nerve (part of vestibulocochlear nerve, or CN VIII) conducts impulses from *organ of Corti in cochlea*
- Fibers originate at spiral ganglion of cochlea, enter anterior surface of brainstem, and travel to posterior and anterior cochlear nuclei
- Impulses from cochlear nuclei ascend through lateral lemniscus, and either terminate in inferior colliculus or pass to *auditory cortex in temporal lobe*

HARDCORE

Herpes simplex viruses (HSV) types 1 and 2 are double-stranded DNA viruses with the following characteristics:

- *Neurovirulence*: The ability to invade neurons and replicate within them
- *Latency*: Maintenance of latent infection within a nerve cell ganglia
- *Reactivation*: Periodic flareups of disease

HARDCORE

The *trigeminal ganglion* is the most common site of latent infection of HSV-1, while the sacral nerve root ganglia are most commonly involved with HSV-2 infection. Viral reactivation often follows a *prodrome of itching and tingling*, and can result in painful vesicle formation on the skin innervated by any of the *branches of the trigeminal nerve* with the associated symptoms of malaise, fever, and lymphadenopathy. Treat with acyclovir.

HARDCORE

Herpes zoster (varicella) is dormant in dorsal root ganglia after initial chickenpox infection. May reactivate as *shingles*. Trigeminal nerve involvement common, with clinical manifestations seen most often in the ophthalmic branch, resulting in *zoster ophthalmicus*, with risk of corneal damage. Symptoms include painful vesicular rash in dermatomal distribution, and *post-herpetic neuralgia*. Treat with high-dose acyclovir.

HARDCORE

Aminoglycoside antibiotics (e.g., gentamicin) interfere with bacterial protein synthesis and are typically used to treat gram-negative infections. They should be used with caution, however, as they can cause *ototoxicity*, resulting in direct damage to the auditory/vestibular system and long-term *hearing loss or balance problems*. *Nephrotoxicity* is also an important side effect.

PATHOLOGIC STATES OF THE SOMATOSENSORY SYSTEM

Peripheral Neuropathies

- *Longer nerves are more susceptible to* damage, resulting in "glove and stocking" distribution of sensory loss, since hands and feet affected first
- Can be caused by a variety of disease states
  - *Diabetes*: Causes ischemic neuropathy presenting with distal sensory loss
  - *Vitamin B and folic acid deficiencies*: Cause demyelinating neuropathy
  - *Alcohol abuse*: Can lead to sensory loss, possibly due to underlying nutritional deficiency
  - *HIV infection*: May cause bilateral foot pain on soles (HIV neuropathy)

Syringomyelia

- Likely due to developmental abnormality in spinal cord; patients develop a "syrinx," or enlargement, of central canal, most often affecting brainstem and cervical region
- Increased risk in patients with *Arnold-Chiari malformation* (downward displacement of cerebellar tonsils into foramen magnum)
- Characteristic signs:
  - *Loss of pain and temperature sensation in shawl-like distribution caused by interruption of lateral spinothalamic tracts as they cross the midline*
  - Ascending tracts of dorsal columns unaffected, resulting in normal tactile discrimination, vibratory sense, and proprioception
  - Horner's syndrome may be present because of interruption of descending autonomic fibers
  - As descending motor tracts become involved, lower motor neuron weakness of hands and bilateral spastic paralysis of legs may occur

CHAPTER 10

Motor Systems

Motor control systems found in higher parts of the brain are responsible for production of complex, goal-directed, and coordinated movements. Roughly divided, there are three major levels of hierarchy of motor control—the cerebral cortex, the brainstem, and the spinal cord (and cranial motor nuclei). Feedback loops and functional interconnections exist between and within each of the three levels. This central axis receives modulatory motor input from the cerebellum and basal ganglia.

CORTICAL MOTOR AREAS

Descending motor commands from cortex project directly to spinal cord, bypassing brainstem, via the **corticospinal tract (CST)**, which carries a large portion of voluntary motor output.

- All located in frontal lobe
- Important source of descending tracts is **primary motor cortex (Brodmann's area 4)**, located anteriorly in the **precentral gyrus**
- Cortical inputs to brainstem travel via **corticobulbar tract**

Primary motor cortex in each hemisphere is organized **somatotopically** (where adjacent cortical areas control adjacent regions of the body) and controls motor function for **contralateral** side of the body.

- Descending motor axons cross the midline at **pyramidal decussation** in the medulla
- **Motor homunculus** schematically represents specific parts of the body, with an orderly progression from most medial (foot/leg) to most lateral portions (head/face), with the trunk of body in between

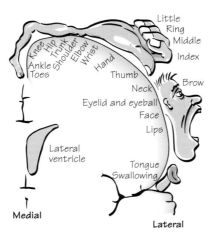

Figure 10-1 Motor homunculus. Cross-sectional view of the primary motor cortex, showing the somatotopic organization where neurons located most medially near the midline control muscles of the lower limb while more lateral portions of the cortex control progressively more rostral parts of the body. The descending axonal tracts from the motor cortex cross the midline in the medulla and descend contralaterally down the spinal cord (not shown). (Modified with permission from Barker RA. Neuroscience at a Glance. 2nd ed. Oxford: Blackwell Publishing, 2003:80.)

- Homunculus is distorted, because the amount of cortex devoted to a muscle group reflects its relative importance
- Blood supply mostly from **middle cerebral artery (MCA)** with contribution from the anterior cerebral aterery (ACA), which supplies the medial portion of the motor cortex
- **Pronator drift** associated with frontal lobe lesions of CST

Premotor cortex (Brodmann's area 6, lateral portion) and **supplementary motor cortex** (Brodmann's area 6, medial portion) thought to be important for motor function that is dependent on sensory input and temporal organization and coordination of complex movements, respectively.

HARDCORE

Because body parts of the homunculus are spread so widely in the motor cortex, cortical strokes are rarely big enough to affect an entire half of the body. Instead, the hands or the face, which take up the most cortical areas, are preferentially affected. In contrast, strokes in the internal capsule tend to paralyze an entire side of the body (resulting in **hemiplegia** or **hemiparesis**), because fibers are bundled closely together. Similarly, if a stroke occurs in the brainstem, affecting the pyramids, the hemiparesis is often accompanied by additional signs such as vertigo, diplopia, or altered consciousness.

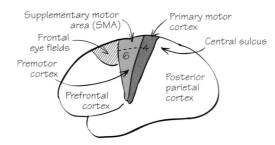

Figure 10-2 **Location of the three motor areas in the precentral gyrus.** (Modified with permission from Barker RA. Neuroscience at a Glance. 2nd ed. Oxford: Blackwell Publishing, 2003:78.)

- Extensive interconnections with primary motor, premotor, somatosensory cortices, basal ganglia, thalamus, and cerebellum
- Lesions associated with **apraxia** (inability to perform motor activities in setting of intact motor and sensory systems)

BRAINSTEM MOTOR AREAS

The brainstem motor areas are the three main regions in humans that serve to integrate visual and vestibular information with somatosensory input to modify movements initiated by the cortex.

Reticular Formation
- Locomotor region located at upper end of midbrain
- Neurons involved in regulation of **arousal**, receive sensory information (limb position, muscle tension) from spinal cord
- Axons form **reticulospinal tract**, involved in spinal reflexes

Vestibular Nuclei
- Located in rostral medulla and caudal pons
- Aids in maintenance of balance and body posture
- Axons sent to cerebellum and reticular motor systems in addition to spinal cord (**vestibulospinal tract**)
- Activation of nuclei promotes limb extension

Red Nucleus
- Located near anterior end of midbrain
- Receives major input from cerebellum
- Sends axons to spinal cord via **rubrospinal tract**, whose activation promotes limb flexion

DESCENDING TRACTS OF THE SPINAL CORD

The spinal cord is the ultimate principal target of output from cortical motor areas.
- Axons originating from each brain motor region travel together in discrete bundles (tracts) that are found in characteristic positions in the white matter of the cord (Figure 10.3)
- Axons from motor cortex form two tracts, the lateral and ventral CST
- Axons from neurons in the red nucleus (rubrospinal) also descend in lateral portion of white matter
- Fibers from vestibular nuclei and reticular formation descend ventrally

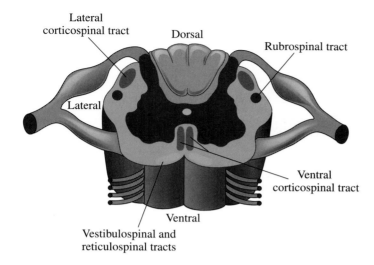

Figure 10-3 Approximate locations in spinal cord white matter of various descending axon tracts from motor control areas in the brain. (Reprinted with permission from Matthews GG. Neurobiology: Molecules, Cells, Systems. 2nd ed. Malden, MA: Blackwell Publishing, 2001:206.)

THE CEREBELLUM AND BASAL GANGLIA

These are two important subcortical processing loops involved in motor control. In general, cerebellar dysfunction is characterized by awkwardness of intentional movements. Lesions of the basal ganglia are often exemplified by meaningless unintentional movements that occur unexpectedly.

Cerebellum

Plays important roles in sensorimotor integration—coordinates information regarding planning and execution of movement of *ipsilateral* side of body. Receives sensory information from spinal cord and vestibular system, then fine-tunes function of descending motor systems to compensate for potential errors. Think sets of threes.

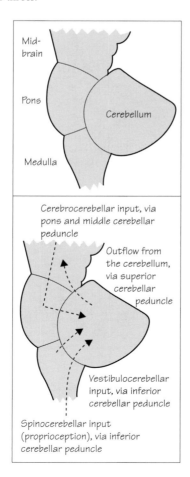

HARDCORE

Cerebellar peduncles:

- Connect cerebellum to brainstem at level of pons
- Superior (primarily output): Contains majority of rostral outflow from cerebellum; fibers continue to lateral ventral thalamus, then to motor cortex via internal capsule; ventral spinocerebellar tract is major afferent pathway
- Middle (primarily input): Consists of fibers from contralateral pontine nuclei
- Inferior (primarily input): Uncrossed ipsilateral inputs from upper and lower extremities that go to both anterior and posterior vermin, and fibers from contralateral inferior olivary nucleus

Figure 10-4 Highly simplified diagram of afferent and efferent pathways between the brainstem and cerebellum. (Reprinted with permission from Wilkinson I. Essential Neurology. 4th ed. Oxford: Blackwell Publishing, 2005:78.)

***Cerebellar cortex*:**

- Molecular layer: Outermost layer, site for synaptic interactions
- Purkinje cell layer: Output to deep nuclei
- Granule layer: Innermost layer, site of mossy fiber input

- Three lobes (flocculonodular, anterior, and posterior)
- Three peduncles (superior, middle, and inferior, through which cerebellar connections pass in or out)
- Three afferent fiber types (mossy from ***spinocerebellar*** pathways, climbing from ***inferior olive nuclei***, aminergic from brainstem)
- Three pairs of deep nuclei
- Three cortical layers
- Located on dorsal aspect of brainstem, posterior to pons and medulla in posterior cranial fossa; forms roof of fourth ventricle
- Receives input from spinal cord and projects to both brainstem and cortex (the latter via the thalamus)

***Cerebellar deep nuclei*:**

- Receives input from cerebellar cortex
- Fastigial: Project to vestibular nuclei and reticular formation (vestibular function)
- Intermediate: Project to red nucleus and thalamus (posture and balance)
- Dentate: Project to thalamus (coordination of extremities)

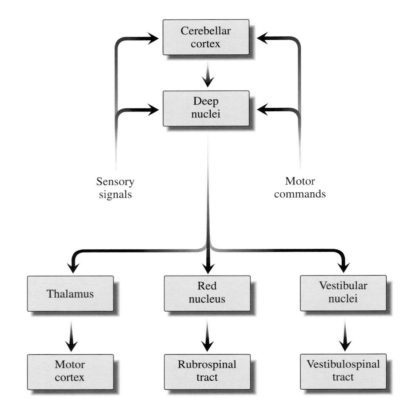

Figure 10-5 Schematic demonstrating major important connections of the cerebellum. (Modified with permission from Matthews GG. Neurobiology: Molecules, Cells, Systems. 2nd ed. Malden, MA: Blackwell Publishing, 2001:206.)

Characteristics of cerebellar lesions:

- Incoordination of muscle activity: Coarse nystagmus and dysarthria (cranial nerves), finger-nose ataxia and dysdiadochokinesia (arms), gait ataxia and heel-knee-shin ataxia (legs)
- Nystagmus worse when looking toward side of lesion
- Decreased tendon reflexes on affected side
- Intention tremor, usually during purposeful movements
- No weakness present (e.g., intoxicated people may have many features of muscular incoordination but remain strong)
- In unilateral cerebellar lesions, neurological deficit is ***ipsilateral*** to side of lesion

- Three functional divisions with distinct anatomical connections to brain and spinal cord
  - Vestibulocerebellum (balance, eye movements)
  - Spinocerebellum (modulates muscle tone and motor execution)
  - Cerebrocerebellum/lateral lobes (motor planning and initiation)

Common causes of cerebellar dysfunction:

- Cerebrovascular disease
- Multiple sclerosis
- Drugs, especially anticonvulsant intoxication
- Acute alcohol intoxication

Rare etiologies of cerebellar dysfunction:

- Posterior fossa neoplasms
- Cerebellar abscess (often secondary to otitis media)
- Cerebellar degeneration, either hereditary (Friedreich's ataxia), alcohol-induced, or paraneoplastic
- Arnold-Chiari malformation
- Hypothyroidism

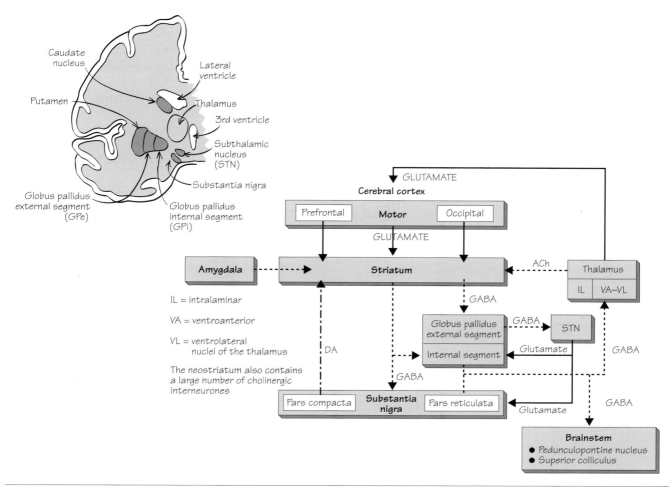

Figure 10-6 Organization of the basal ganglia, showing functional grouping of the extensively interconnected nuclei. The substantia nigra is located in the midbrain. Solid lines represent excitatory input, while dashed lines represent inhibitory input. (Modified with permission from Barker RA. Neuroscience at a Glance. 2nd ed. Oxford: Blackwell Publishing, 2003:84.)

Basal Ganglia

Consists of three interconnected groups of subcortical neurons—*caudate nucleus*, *putamen*, and *globus pallidus*—found in the central portion of the telencephalon. *Subthalamic nucleus* and *substantia nigra* are sometimes grouped together as well. All are involved in motor control. Together, the caudate nucleus and the putamen are known as the *striatum*, while the globus pallidus and the putamen are referred to as *lentiform nuclei*.

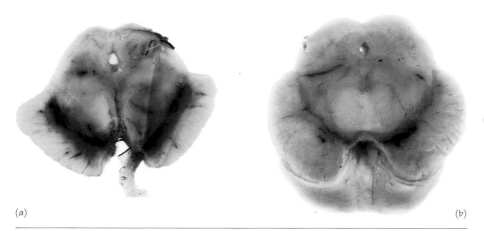

(a)   (b)

Figure 10-7 Gross cross-sections of substantia nigra in normal (a) and Parkinson's (b) patients demonstrating loss of pigment in the latter. (Reprinted with permission from Ginsberg L. Lecture Notes: Neurology. 8th ed. Oxford: Blackwell Publishing, 2005:93.)

HARDCORE

Parkinsonism is a degenerative syndrome primarily affecting extrapyramidal pathways where dopamine is the neurotransmitter, and is characterized by the clinical triad of akinesia, *"cogwheel" rigidity*, and resting *"pill-rolling"* or *"head-nodding" tremor*. Other features include stooped posture, diminished facial expression ("masked facies"), and *shuffling ("festinant") gait*. Most commonly found after damage to *substantia nigra* and its projections to the striatum, most famously after exposure to *MPTP* (synthetic heroin byproduct); etiologies neither hereditary nor infectious.

HARDCORE

Parkinson's disease (PD) is common, affecting 1% to 2% of population aged 60+ years. *Lewy bodies* are seen in the melanin-containing neurons microscopically, and contribute to symptoms of dementia. Progressive supranuclear palsy often occurs. Disease is progressive, and current therapies aim to correct the *dopamine deficiency (levodopa/carbidopa)* and relieve symptoms. Surgical intervention possible for advanced cases.

HARDCORE

Huntington's disease (HD) is a disease primarily affecting the caudate and putamen with age of onset in the early 40s. It is an **autosomal dominant** disorder caused by an **expanded trinucleotide CAG repeat** at a single gene. Disease also demonstrates **anticipation** —symptoms tend to become progressively worse and present at an earlier age with each generation, as the expanded repeats become longer.

HARDCORE

Degeneration of the caudate and putamen in HD results in decreased GABAergic inhibition, producing continuous dance-like movements of the face and limbs (**chorea**), sudden jerky unintentional movements, and writhing, snakelike movements (**athetosis**). Motor problems usually accompanied by behavioral changes and progressive dementia. Pathologically, there is atrophy of the caudate, along with more generalized cerebral atrophy (frontal and temporal lobes). HD is relentless, with death ensuing within 15 years.

HARDCORE

In **hemiballismus**, a disorder related to HD, flailing, violent, and jerky movements of proximal muscles in the extremities restricted to one side of the body (unilateral ballism), occurring as a result of damage (vascular lesions such as stroke) to the contralateral **subthalamic nucleus**.

HARDCORE

Wilson's disease (hepatolenticular degeneration) is a rare autosomal recessive defect of **copper metabolism**. Levels of serum copper and its transporter protein ceruloplasmin are low, and copper is deposited most commonly in the liver, basal ganglia (**lentiform nucleus**), and limbus of cornea (**Kayser-Fleischer rings**). Neurological features include an akinetic-rigid syndrome, tremors, dystonia, cerebellar signs, and neuropsychiatric manifestations including psychosis. Mainstay of treatment is **penicillamine**, a copper chelator.

- Receives inputs from motor cortex and projects back to it indirectly via parts of thalamus; essential for motor control and refinement of movements
- No direct connections with either spinal cord or brainstem motor systems
- Substantia nigra contains high concentrations of **dopamine**, which oxidizes to form the classic dark pigment seen in fresh brain sections; GABA is main transmitter in projections to thalamus
- Lesions produce characteristic motor deficits
  ○ **Hypokinesia**: Characterized by impairment in initiating movements **(akinesia)** and reduction in amplitude and velocity of voluntary movements **(bradykinesia)**
  ○ **Hyperkinesia**: Characterized by excessive motor activity in the form of involuntary movements and varying degrees of hypotonia

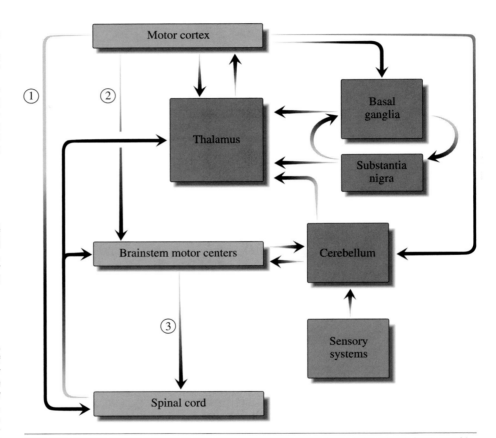

Figure 10-8 Summary of the interconnections of the major motor control systems. Arrow 1 is the corticospinal tract, arrow 2 is the corticobulbar tract, and arrow 3 represents the reticulospinal, vestibulospinal, and rubrospinal tracts. The cortex is connected to the cerebellum indirectly through the brainstem relay nuclei. (Modified with permission from Matthews GG. Neurobiology: Molecules, Cells, Systems. 2nd ed. Malden, MA: Blackwell Publishing, 2001:207.)

CHAPTER 11

Higher Functions and the Limbic System

The limbic system is composed of a complex set of structures that lie above and around the thalamus, just under the cerebrum. It includes the hypothalamus, the hippocampus, the amygdala, and several neighboring areas with intricate and often looped connections. These structures have been implicated in a wide variety of behavioral and emotional functions. Along with the Papez circuit, the limbic system also appears to be critical for remembering and learning.

BASIC ANATOMY AND MAJOR STRUCTURES

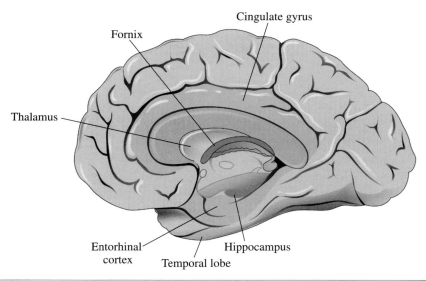

Figure 11-1 Organization of the limbic system. Diagram of major components of limbic system. (Reprinted with permission from Matthews GG. Neurobiology: Molecules, Cells, Systems. 2nd ed. Malden, MA: Blackwell Publishing, 2001:262.)

Orbitofrontal Cortex
- Mediates conscious perception of smell
- Projects to cingulated gyrus
- Lesions here cause behavioral problems such as *disinhibition, impulsivity, and emotional lability*

Cingulate Gyrus
- Curves around corpus callosum in each cerebral hemisphere
- Has many connections with anterior thalamic nuclei
- Coordinates sensory input with emotions
- Hyperactivity in cingulate gyrus associated with *Tourette's syndrome*

Thalamus
- Mediodorsal nucleus has connections with prefrontal cortex and hypothalamus
- Anterior nucleus connects with the mammillary bodies and cingulate gyrus

- *Serves as "relay station" for auditory, visual, and somatic input to cortex*
- Thalamic lesions can result in loss of somatic sensation, pain syndromes (from disruption of sensory input), thalamic aphasia, and behavioral changes

Entorhinal Cortex

- Anterior portion of parahippocampal gyrus
- Receives cognitive and sensory information from association areas and relays to *hippocampal formation* for consolidation

Hypothalamus

Important in *control of autonomic nervous system (ANS)*, maintenance of *homeostasis* in many physiological systems, control of *circadian and endocrine functions*, and formation of *anterograde memory*.

- Organization:
  - Forms floor of *third ventricle*
  - Most ventral portion has *median eminence*, from which the *infundibulum* (pituitary stalk) arises
  - Composed of many different nuclei: anterior, tuberal, and posterior

ANTERIOR HYPOTHALAMIC NUCLEI

- Monitor serum osmolality via *osmoreceptors in lamina terminalis*
- Produce *oxytocin and antidiuretic hormone (ADH)* (stored in posterior pituitary gland)
- Regulate autonomic function via projections from *paraventricular nuclei*
- Help regulate sleep/circadian rhythms via *suprachiasmatic nucleus*

TUBERAL HYPOTHALAMIC NUCLEI

- Central portion of hypothalamus important for feeding, emotional behavior, and endocrine function
- **Lesion of lateral nuclei results in anorexia/weight loss**
- *Dorsomedial and ventromedial nuclei involved in satiety*

POSTERIOR HYPOTHALAMIC NUCLEI

- Involved in temperature regulation, limbic function, and memory functions
- Contain *mammillary bodies*, which receive input from hippocampal formation
  - Medial mammillary nuclei project to thalamus along mamillothalamic tract (part of Papez circuit)
  - Lateral mammillary nuclei project to nuclei in midbrain and pons

Hippocampal Formation

- Major functions are *learning and memory*
- Consists of *hippocampus* itself, *dentate gyrus*, and *subiculum*
- Receives *afferents* primarily from *inferior temporal cortex* via *entorhinal cortex*
- Sends *efferents* from hippocampus and subiculum via *fornix* to *mammillary bodies* of hypothalamus

DENTATE GYRUS

- Main input area of hippocampal formation
- Contains granule cells that receive input

HIPPOCAMPUS

- Two "horns" that curve back from the area of the hypothalamus to the amygdala
- Located in medial temporal lobe
- Contains pyramidal cells that project to septal area and hypothalamus
- Main processing area of hippocampal formation

SUBICULUM

- Main output area
- Continuous with entorhinal cortex

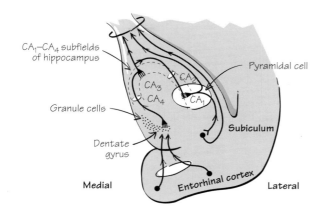

Figure 11-2 Simplified schematic of hippocampus anatomy. (Modified with permission from Barker RA. Neuroscience at a Glance. 2nd ed. Oxford: Blackwell Publishing, 2003:84.)

Amygdala

- Bilateral groups of nuclei in antero-inferior region of temporal lobe
- Involved with emotions such as love, fear, rage, and aggression
- Connects with hippocampus, septal nuclei, prefrontal area, and medial dorsal nucleus of thalamus

Septal Nuclei

- Interconnected with amygdala and hypothalamus
- Implicated in modulation of sexual pleasure and maternal behavior

HARDCORE

The hippocampus is divided into four fields, designated CA-1 through CA-4. *CA-1 (Sommer's sector) is particularly susceptible to damage* secondary to ischemia, hypoxia, or hypoglycemia. This is termed *selective vulnerability*. Sommer's sector is also considered a *trigger zone* for seizures in *temporal lobe epilepsy*.

HARDCORE

Klüver-Bucy syndrome results from bilateral *ablation of medial temporal lobes*, including *amygdaloid nuclei*. Symptoms include:

- Psychic blindness (visual agnosia)
- Hypersexuality
- Hyperorality
- Passivity

HARDCORE

Papez circuit is a historically defined group of interconnected neurons that serves as the structural core of the limbic system.

- Includes hippocampal formation, mammillary bodies, thalamus, cingulate gyrus
- Circuit demonstrates the interconnectivity of the cortex and hypothalamus

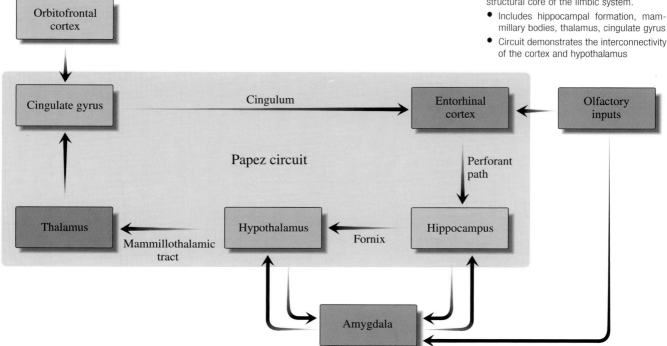

Figure 11-3 Papez circuit. (Reprinted with permission from Matthews GG. Neurobiology: Molecules, Cells, Systems. 2nd ed. Malden, MA: Blackwell Publishing, 2001:262.)

Long-term potentiation (LTP):

- Defined as increase in strength of synaptic transmission
- Mediated by excitatory glutamate synapses containing NMDA receptors

Dopamine-secreting neurons from the *ventral tegmental area* and the *limbic system* form the *mesolimbic dopaminergic pathway*. These neurons send input to the *nucleus accumbens*, and are responsible for sensation of pleasure. This pathway is involved in functions ranging from motivation and reward to feeding and drug addiction.

TYPES OF MEMORY

- *Anterograde*: Acquisition of new material
- *Retrograde*: Recall of previously learned information
- *Short-term*: Working memory for immediate recall
- *Long-term*
  - *Explicit* (declarative): Concerned with learned facts
    - E.g., episodic memory (result of personal experience)
    - E.g., semantic memory (result of education)
    - Bilateral temporal lobectomy results in severely impaired explicit memory and anterograde amnesia
  - *Implicit* (procedural): Concerned with learned motor responses
    - Structures involved include dominant parietal cortex, cerebellum, basal ganglia, and frontal association cortex
- *Long-term potentiation* of granule and pyramidal neurons in the *hippocampus is key in memory acquisition and consolidation* (converting short-term to long-term memory)

CHAPTER 12

Paroxysmal Disorders

Paroxysmal disorders are characterized by their intermittent nature. Patients are clinically normal between attacks, and episodes can occur with varying frequencies. In this chapter, seizures, headache, and common sleep disorders are discussed.

SEIZURES

- Transient cerebral dysfunction caused by abnormal neuronal discharge
- Broadly classified as *generalized* or *partial*

Primary Generalized

- Entire brain involved
- Two major types, tonic-clonic and absence

Tonic-Clonic (Grand Mal)

- Attack may be preceded by dizziness or irritability
- *Tonic* phase: Sustained tonic contraction of muscles with whole body stiffening, usually in extended position; patient is not breathing during this phase but may let out *epileptic cry* as air is forced from lungs
- *Clonic* phase: Strong, random, repetitive jerking movements following tonic phase

Absence (Petit Mal)

- Onset usually between 4–8 years; girls affected more commonly
- Child stares into space during attack; eyes may roll back
- May have hundreds of attacks per day
- 10% risk of continued seizures into adulthood

Partial

- Dysfunction begins in focal area of brain
- May or may not generalize and is often preceded by aura

Simple Partial

- No loss of consciousness during seizure
- May involve motor, sensory, or autonomic systems (e.g., strong convulsive movement or sensation in limb, face, or part of body)

Complex Partial (Temporal Lobe, Psychomotor)

- Consciousness impaired
- Patient may experience aura before attack: Fear; déjà vu; olfactory, gustatory, or visual hallucinations; confusion; anxiousness; or automatisms (stereotyped behaviors)

Partial Seizures with Secondary Generalization

- Aberrant neuronal firing during partial seizure may progress from one cortical area to the next, a process termed *Jacksonian march*
- *Todd's paralysis*: Temporary weakness in affected limbs following seizure

Benign Febrile Convulsions of Childhood

- Typically generalized seizures triggered by *fevers*
- Occur in 3% of children between 3 months and 5 years of age

HARDCORE

Status epilepticus: Seizures that occur for *more than 30 minutes*, with such frequency that *patient does not regain consciousness between episodes*. This is a MEDICAL EMERGENCY that can result in permanent brain damage secondary to *anoxia, hyperpyrexia, circulatory collapse, or excitotoxic neuronal damage*. Causes include lack of adherence to anti-seizure medications, alcohol (lowers seizure threshold), trauma, CNS infections, tumor, stroke, hypoxia, hypoglycemia, and drug overdose (e.g., antidepressants).

HARDCORE

Treatment for status epilepticus:

- *Ensure that airway is patent*, and that patient is positioned to prevent aspiration
- Begin anticonvulsants immediately:
  - Lorazepam or diazepam
  - Phenytoin
  - If seizures persist, give phenobarbital
  - If seizures persist, proceed to general anesthesia
- Give dextrose
- Laboratory studies, including lumbar puncture if patient has fever or meningeal signs

TABLE 12-1 Common Causes of New-Onset Seizures

PRIMARY NEUROLOGIC DISORDERS	SYSTEMIC DISORDERS
• Benign febrile convulsions of childhood • Idiopathic epilepsy • Head trauma • Stroke • Mass lesions • Meningitis or encephalitis • HIV encephalopathy	• Hypoglycemia • Hyponatremia • Hyperosmolar states • Hypocalcemia • Uremia • Hepatic encephalopathy • Porphyria • Drug overdose or withdrawal • Global cerebral ischemia • Eclampsia • Hyperthermia • Hypertensive encephalopathy

TABLE 12-2 Common Causes of Seizures by Age Group

NEONATES	CHILDREN	YOUNG ADULTS	MIDDLE-AGED	ELDERLY
• Birth trauma • Intracranial hemorrhage • Hypoxia • Hypoglycemia • Hypocalcemia	• Congenital anomalies • Tuberous sclerosis • Metabolic storage diseases	• Head injury • Drugs/alcohol intoxication and withdrawal	• Cerebral tumor	• Cerebrovascular disease • Degenerative disorders (Alzheimer's, prion disease)

HARDCORE

Know the common causes of seizures listed in Table 12.2

- Occur as isolated attack in 70% of cases
- Generally do not require long-term anticonvulsant therapy
- Table 12.1 lists common causes of new-onset seizures
- Table 12.2 lists common causes of seizures by age group

Seizure Treatment

Usually, antiepileptic drugs are not started after a single isolated seizure, especially if secondary to a treatable condition such as meningitis or alcohol withdrawal.

Anticonvulsants

- Most are *membrane stabilizers* that limit firing of action potentials
- Use dose that prevents seizures ("therapeutic serum level")
- Upper limit determined by side effects, which include drowsiness
- Cerebellar syndromes (slurred speech and ataxia), teratogenicity

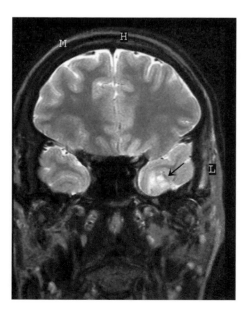

Figure 12-1 Coronal MRI of brain showing developmental abnormality of temporal lobe (arrow) that acted as an epileptogenic focus. (Reprinted with permission from Ginsberg L. Lecture Notes: Neurology. 8th ed. Oxford: Blackwell Publishing, 2005:78.)

○ *Gingival hyperplasia, acne, hirsutism (phenytoin)*

○ *Alopecia, elevated liver function tests (LFTs) (valproate)*

- *Restrictions on driving* and certain activities may be necessary in those with uncontrolled epilepsy

- Patients in whom a *highly focal* region of the brain causes seizures may benefit from *surgical removal of epileptogenic focus*

HEADACHES

Range in etiology from benign to life threatening. Characteristic patient symptoms (onset, duration, and distribution) often offer keys to diagnosis.

Tension Headache

- Described as *tight band around head (non-throbbing, bilateral)*
- Poor response to analgesics
- Often *stress-related* or due to rebound secondary to sudden cessation of chronic analgesic use

Migraine

- *Throbbing* pain, usually *unilateral*
- Associated with *photophobia, nausea, vomiting*
- May be accompanied by *flashing lights, blurred vision, speech disturbance, or sensory symptoms*
- More common in *females*
- Familial predisposition
- *Triggers:*
  ○ *Certain foods, hunger*
  ○ *Alcohol*
  ○ *Menstruation*
  ○ *Stress, physical activity*
  ○ *Oral contraceptives*
- Etiology unknown; may be vascular or neurogenic
- Treatments include *analgesics*, serotonergic agents (*sumatriptan*), antiemetics, alkaloids (*ergotamine*)
- Prophylactic treatments include beta-blockers (propanolol), anticonvulsants, serotonin agonists, calcium-channel blockers, tricyclic antidepressants

Cluster Headache (Migrainous Neuralgia)

- *Severe, stabbing, intermittent pain* occurring repetitively over weeks with long pain-free intervals between episodes (often months)
- More common in *males*
- Pain often located in *orbit*, accompanied by redness, swelling, unilateral nasal congestion, and lacrimation
- Prophylaxis includes *analgesics* and *ergotamine*

Trigeminal Neuralgia (Tic Douloureux)

- Sudden, transient, stabbing pain recurring several times a day
- Usually *unilateral in distribution of maxillary or mandibular branch of trigeminal nerve (CN 5)*
- Triggers include *cold wind, touching face, brushing teeth, talking, chewing*
- Usually affects patients > 50 years old
- Etiology often idiopathic, but may be secondary to *compression of trigeminal nerve* (neuroma, meningioma, aberrant arterial loop) or *multiple sclerosis* (demyelination in brainstem)
- Treatment includes anticonvulsants (carbamazepine or phenytoin) or surgical ablation

Elevated Intracranial Pressure (ICP)

- Can result from *space-occupying lesions (neoplasm, abscess, hematoma)*
- Associated headache is *present on awakening*
- Pain exacerbated by *sneezing, straining, bending, lifting, and lying down* (anything that further increases intracranial pressure)

HARDCORE

Subarachnoid hemorrhage (SAH): *"Worst headache of my life."* Bleeding into the subarachnoid space secondary to *ruptured aneurysm*, arteriovenous malformation, trauma, coagulopathies results in *very sudden onset pain (within seconds)* due to meningeal irritation. Patients may also have *photophobia, nausea, vomiting, neck stiffness, depressed consciousness,* and *papilledema*. Management includes immediate resuscitation, CT scan, lumbar puncture (if mass lesion ruled out), cerebral angiography to permit clipping of aneurysm. High mortality with high risk of rebleeding.

HARDCORE

Temporal arteritis (giant cell arteritis):

- *Arteritis of extracranial and intraorbital arteries*; vessels show *granulomatous* changes and narrowing of lumen

- *Occlusion of vessels to optic nerve threatens vision*

- Occurs in *elderly patients*

- Symptoms include *headache and scalp tenderness* (e.g., upon combing hair), transient loss of vision in one eye (*amaurosis fugax*)

- Constitutional symptoms (fever, malaise, night sweats, anorexia, weight loss) often present

- *Superficial temporal artery* may be *tender, red, swollen,* and *nonpulsatile*

- Viral or autoimmune etiology suspected

- Treat with *high-dose intravenous steroids*; diagnosis by *temporal artery biopsy* and *elevated erythrocyte sedimentation rate (ESR)*

- Associated with polymyalgia rheumatica

- Other symptoms include *papilledema, dimished consciousness, vomiting, and focal neurologic signs secondary to space-occupying lesion*
- Lumbar puncture may be therapeutic; however, *in setting of mass lesion, sudden release of pressure may result in brain herniation*
- Treatment includes intubation, *hyperventilation* (since elevated carbon dioxide causes cerebral vessel dilatation and increased pressure), and *mannitol*

SLEEP DISORDERS

Unlike coma, sleep is a state of unconsciousness from which a person can be aroused. The *sleep-wake cycle* depends on the intrinsic rhythm of the *reticular activating system (RAS)*.

Narcolepsy
- Condition of irresistible attacks of sudden sleep that occur at any time
- Tetrad of clinical features:
  - **Uncontrollable sleep attacks and overwhelming daytime sleepiness**
  - *Cataplexy*
    - Loss of postural control with maintained consciousness
    - Can be provoked by emotional events and stress
  - *Sleep paralysis*
    - Inability to move while falling asleep or waking up
  - *Hypnagogic hallucinations*
    - Visual hallucinations while falling asleep

Sleep Apnea

OBSTRUCTIVE
- Upper airway obstruction during sleep that results in apneic episodes
- Under-recognized cause of daytime somnolence
- Associated with *obesity*
- May result in *pulmonary hypertension*
- Can be treated by weight loss, use of continuous positive airway pressure (CPAP) at night, or surgery to correct underlying anatomical abnormalities

CENTRAL
- Less common
- Apneic epsidoes without obstruction
- Occurs in patients with severe and life-threatening *lower brainstem lesions* (secondary to bulbar poliomyelitis, encephalitis, stroke, radiation, surgery, and neurodegenerative disorders)

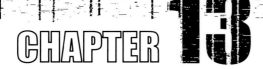

CHAPTER 13

Cerebrospinal Fluid and Central Nervous System Infections

The CNS is susceptible to infection by bacteria, viruses, fungi, parasites, and other agents. Many infections lead to atypical alterations in the cerebrospinal fluid (CSF) and characteristic signs and symptoms. In this chapter, normal production and function of the CSF is discussed along with manifestations of common CNS infections.

MENINGES

The meninges are **three connective tissue membranes** that line the spinal cord and the brain. Starting from the brain and moving outward, the three layers are:

- **Pia mater** (which hugs the brain)
- **Arachnoid mater** (pia mater and arachnoid make up the "**leptomeninges**")
- **Dura mater**
- Between the pia mater and the arachnoid is the **subarachnoid space** (think "below the arachnoid"), where cerebrospinal fluid (CSF) is found.

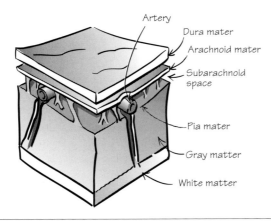

Figure 13-1 **Relationship between meninges and brain tissue.** (Modified with permission from Barker RA. Neuroscience at a Glance. 2nd ed. Oxford: Blackwell Publishing, 2003:40.)

LUMBAR PUNCTURE

Indications for Lumbar Puncture

EMERGENT INDICATIONS

- **Suspected acute bacterial meningitis**
- **CNS infections**
- **Subarachnoid hemorrhage**

OTHER DIAGNOSTIC INDICATIONS

- Chronic CNS infections (tuberculous and fungal meningitis, neurosyphilis)
- Demyelinating disease
- Other inflammatory disease (e.g., vasculitis)

Contraindications for Lumbar Puncture

- *Infection near puncture site*
- *Cranial or spinal mass on CT (to avoid herniation)*
- *Bleeding diathesis*

Anatomy

- In adults, the spinal cord extends to the lower borders of L1–L2. To avoid damage to the cord, the needle is usually placed between *L3 and L4 or L4 and L5*. Note: In neonates, the conus medullaris extends to L3.
- Layers passed through during insertion of the needle:
  1. Skin/superficial fascia
  2. Ligaments (supraspinous, interspinous, ligamentum flavum)
  3. Epidural space
  4. Dura mater
  5. Subdural space
  6. Arachnoid mater
  7. Subarachnoid space (where CSF is contained)

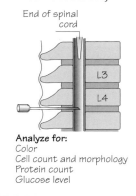

Analyze for:
Color
Cell count and morphology
Protein count
Glucose level

Figure 13-2 Anatomy passed through during lumbar puncture. (Modified with permission from Barker RA. Neuroscience at a Glance. 2nd ed. Oxford: Blackwell Publishing, 2003:106.)

VENTRICULAR SYSTEM

The ventricles contain CSF and are lined by *choroid plexus*, a specialized vascular structure that *makes and secretes CSF*.

- The foramen of Munro connects the two lateral ventricles to the third ventricle
- The cerebral aqueduct connects the third ventricle to the fourth ventricle
- The fourth ventricle connects to the subarachnoid space via three foramina: Mnemonic: "**LLMM**"—Two Lateral foramina of Luschka, and the Midline foramen of Magendie

CSF Production, Reabsorption, and Function

- CSF is produced at a rate of 22 cc per hour, or 0.5 liter per day
- CSF circulates in the subarachnoid space through the ventricular system, around the brain and spinal cord, and eventually is reabsorbed by the *arachnoid granulations*. The total volume of CSF in an adult is about 150 cc
- CSF cushions the brain and spinal cord, providing protection against trauma
- Composition similar to blood plasma, but CSF contains less albumin and glucose

INFECTIONS OF THE CENTRAL NERVOUS SYSTEM

Inflammation of the leptomeninges is commonly known as *meningitis*.

Acute Bacterial Meningitis

- Two-thirds of adult patients present with the classic clinical triad of fever, neck stiffness, and headache/altered mental status. *Neck stiffness is rare in elderly and neonates*
- Predisposing factors for acute bacterial meningitis

HARDCORE

Hydrocephalus can be defined broadly as a disturbance of the formation, flow, or absorption of CSF that leads to an *increase in volume* of this fluid in the central nervous system. Mechanistically, a disconnection between the site of CSF production (choroids plexus in the cerebral ventricles) and its site of absorption (arachnoid villi contiguous with subarachnoid space) results in *ventricular dilatation*. Patients present with headache, nausea, vomiting, decreased level of consciousness, papilledema, and sixth nerve palsies.

HARDCORE

Two general classifications of hydrocephalus:

- *Obstructive/noncommunicating*: Typically refers to hydrocephalus that develops as a result of blockage in normal circulation of CSF within the brain. Acute obstructive hydrocephalous requires urgent removal of excess CSF via a *ventricular drain*, or, as a more permanent measure, *ventriculoperitoneal shunting*. In most cases there is a blockage between the third and fourth ventricles (*aqueductal obstruction*). May result from:
  - Congenital abnormalities (cerebral aqueduct stenosis, Arnold-Chiari malformation)
  - Mass lesions (tumor, hematoma)
- *Communicating*: If CSF flow is blocked "beyond" the ventricular system (e.g., as a result of damage to the meninges and obstruction of the arachnoid villi). Causes include:
  - Meningitis
  - Subarachnoid hemorrhage (may also cause obstructive hydrocephalus)
  - Increased CSF viscosity

HARDCORE

Signs and symptoms of meningitis:
- Fever
- Headache
- Nuchal rigidity ("stiff neck")
- Nausea/vomiting
- Mental status alterations
- Photophobia

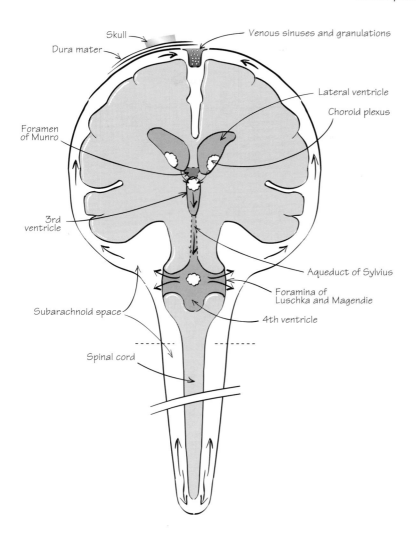

Figure 13-3 Coronal section of brain showing path of CSF from ventricles to subarachnoid space. CSF flows through the ventricular system as follows: It is generated in the choroids plexus, passes through lateral ventricles, enters the third ventricle via the interventricular foramina of Monro, enters the fourth ventricle via the cerebral aqueduct of Sylvius, and finally enters the subarachnoid space via either the foramen of Luschka (lateral) or Magendie (medial). (Modified with permission from Barker RA. Neuroscience at a Glance. 2nd ed. Oxford: Blackwell Publishing, 2003:40.)

○ Age (>50 y)

○ Immunodeficiency (asplenia, chemotherapy, HIV)

○ Chronic diseases (diabetes mellitus, cirrhosis, alcoholism)

○ Infection (tuberculosis, sinusitis, pneumonia, otitis media)

○ Open head or spine trauma

○ Table 13-1 lists the causes of acute bacterial meningitis

HARDCORE

Know the causes of acute bacterial meningitis listed in Table 13-1.

TABLE 13-1	Causes of Acute Bacterial Meningitis		
NEWBORNS (< 6 MONTHS)	INFANTS AND YOUNG CHILDREN	YOUNG ADULTS	OLDER ADULTS (60+)
Group B *Streptococcus*	*Streptococcus pneumoniae*	*Neisseria meningitidis*	*Streptococcus pneumoniae*
Escherichia coli	*Neisseria meningitidis*	*Streptococcus pneumoniae*	*Listeria monocytogenes*
Listeria monocytogenes	*Haemophilus influenzae* (decreased incidence secondary to vaccination)		

TB meningitis infections in immunocompromised patients:
- Result from infection with *Mycobacterium tuberculosis*
- Typically has a slower course than bacterial meningitis, with more vasculitic effect resulting in *ischemia and stroke*
- Include these clinical features: Persistent headache, fever, seizures, focal neurological signs
- May result in **chronic caseating granulomas**
- In the form of spinal tuberculosis, can cause cord compression (**Pott's disease of the spine**)
- Is treated with triple/quadruple antimycobacterial therapy

Cerebral toxoplasmosis infections in immunocompromised patients:
- Result from infection with *Toxoplasma gondii* (a single-celled parasite)
- May be acquired via cat feces, undercooked meat, or contaminated water
- Include these signs and symptoms: Focal hemispheric, cerebellar or cranial nerve deficits, headache, seizures, encephalitis, or birth defects

CNS cryptococcosis infections in immunocompromised patients:
- Result in meningoencephalitis caused by **encapsulated** yeast *Cryptococcus neoformans* (often found in soil contaminated with bird droppings); acquired by inhalation
- Has AIDS as major risk factor for infection
- Commonly has symptoms including headache, altered mental status, confusion, lethargy, obtundation, coma
- Diagnosed by capsule visualized with **India ink stain**

Know the CSF profiles listed in Table 13-2.

Caused by infection with the spirochete *Treponema pallidum*, **neurosyphilis** has seen an increase in the last decade, mostly in patients with concomitant **HIV infection**. Manifestations can include **tabes dorsalis** (paresthesias, loss of proprioceptive and vibratory sensation) and the **Argyll-Robertson pupil** (loss of pupillary reaction to light with preservation of constriction to accommodation). Most patients will have a **positive VDRL** and/or elevated lymphocytes and protein in the CSF. Treatment: **Penicillin G**.

Subacute sclerosing panencephalitis is a rare, fatal degenerative CNS disorder resulting from infection with **mutant measles virus**. Patients usually have **normal recovery from initial measles infection**, only to develop **neurological symptoms 2–10 years later**. Symptoms include behavioral changes, myoclonic jerking, seizures, dementia, ataxia; typical wave pattern on EEG present. Disease usually occurs in children and adolescents, and results from direct invasion of brain cells by measles virus, resulting in **encephalitis**.

- Acute bacterial meningitis is a **MEDICAL EMERGENCY**. If CT imaging is felt to be necessary before performing a lumbar puncture (LP), obtain blood cultures and start empiric antibiotics promptly. Do LP as soon as possible after CT. Complications of acute bacterial meningitis include seizures, cranial neuropathies, cerebral edema, hydrocephalus, herniation, infarcts, and death
- Close contacts of patients with meningococcal meningitis should receive **prophylaxis**: **Rifampin or ciprofloxacin**

Viral (Aseptic) Meningitis

- Named for inability to grow pathogen out of CSF
- Less fulminant than acute bacterial meningitis, with spontaneous recovery within weeks
- Presents with meningeal signs plus focal neural deficits and seizures
- Commonly associated viruses include enteroviruses (mumps, coxsackievirus, echovirus), Epstein-Barr virus (EBV), and herpes simplex virus 2 (HSV-2).

Brain Abscess

- Presents as an expanding intracranial mass lesion like a brain tumor, with signs of meningismus plus focal neurological symptoms. Fever and increased white count not always present
- Common organisms include *Staphylococcus aureus*, *Streptococcus*, Enterobacteriaceae, and, rarely, *Bacteroides* and *Nocardia*; *Toxoplasma* in HIV; *Taenia solium* (causing cysticercosis) in underdeveloped countries. Multiple organisms often present. Epidural abscess (staph, strep, gram-negative rods, anaerobes) can occur, especially in the spinal canal, and requires surgical drainage and antibiotics
- Risk factors include **IV drug use**, **endocarditis**, trauma, dental infections

Viral Encephalitis

- Encephalitis results from viral infection of brain parenchyma. Patients present with psychotic behavior, confusion, headache, fever, meningeal signs, and seizures
- **HSV-1** and, to a lesser degree, HSV-2 are the most common culprits and often affect the limbic cortex. Virus identified via PCR. Classic MRI findings are **unilateral or bilateral temporal and frontal lobe necrosis**. **Acyclovir** is essential to prevent **coma and death**

Lyme Disease

- Caused by infection with spirochete *Borrelia burgdorferi*, transmitted via tick bite
- Acute phase includes **fever**, **rash**, **joint pains**, meningism
- Chronic phase (weeks/months after tick bite) may include meningitis, encephalitis, **cranial nerve palsies** (**facial nerve most commonly affected**), spinal root and peripheral nerve lesions.
- Treatment: Ceftriaxone

TABLE 13-2	**CSF Profiles**				
	APPEARANCE	**PROTEIN**	**GLUCOSE**	**CELLS**	**OTHER**
Normal	Clear	0.1–0.4 g/L	About 50% serum value	< 5 leukocytes/µL	
Acute bacterial meningitis	Clear to turbid, colorless to xanthochromic*	↑↑	↓ to ↓↓	↑ to ↑↑ (polymorphonuclear cells)	70% positive cultures
Aseptic or viral meningitis	Clear, colorless	Normal to ↑	Normal	↑ (lymphocytes, monocytes)	Viral cultures rarely positive
Acute viral encephalitis	Clear to slightly turbid, xanthochromic* in HSV	Normal to ↑	Normal to ↓	↑ (lymphocytes, monocytes)	HSV PCR useful
Fungal meningitis	Clear to cloudy	↑	Normal to ↓	↑ (lymphocytes, polymorphonuclear cells)	
TB meningitis	Cloudy	↑	↓	↑ (lymphocytes, polymorphonuclear cells)	Slow to culture

* Xanthochromic refers to yellow spinal fluid, most commonly due to metabolized blood from subarachnoid hemorrhage. Other agents causing lymphocyte-predominant meningitides include syphilis and CNS Lyme disease.

CHAPTER 14

Space-Occupying Lesions

Space-occupying lesions such as tumors and bleeds are especially important in the context of the limited physical space inside the cranium. Neoplasia in the CNS can be broadly divided into either benign or malignant lesions. Intracranial tumors are further classified into primary (neoplasms arising in neuromuscular tissues themselves) or secondary/metastatic (neoplasms that spread in the circulation from other primary organ sites). It is important to become familiar with the presumed cell of origin, preferential location, most common age group affected, pattern of growth, clinical signs/symptoms, prognosis, and therapies of the major types of brain tumors. Intracranial bleeds and hematomas are favorite exam topics, thus mastery of the key characteristics is essential.

INTRACRANIAL COMPARTMENTS AND INCREASED INTRACRANIAL PRESSURE (ICP)

Dura, falx cerebri, and tentorium cerebelli divide space within skull into three large compartments.

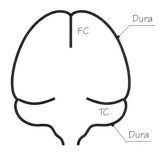

Figure 14-1 The rigid frame containing the brain and its major compartments. FC, falx cerebri; TC, tentorium cerebelli. (Reprinted with permission from Wilkinson I. Essential Neurology. 4th ed. Oxford: Blackwell Publishing, 2005:41.)

- One cerebral hemisphere above each tentorium cerebelli, with cerebellum and brainstem below (in posterior fossa)
- Increased cranial pressure results in distortion and displacement of brain matter downward and toward the foramen magnum
- Signs include headache, vomiting, blurred vision, and *papilledema*

BRAIN TUMORS

Categorized as benign (generally extra-axial, arising from meninges or CNs) or malignant (generally intra-axial, arising from within brain parenchyma).

- Primary brain tumors arise from CNS tissue, account for more than half of all cases of adult intracranial neoplasms, and are commonly of glial cell origin (*gliomas*)
- Remainder of brain neoplasms caused by metastatic cancer originating outside the CNS (in order of decreasing frequency—carcinomas of the lung, breast, ovary, gastrointestinal tract, melanoma, and kidney)
- In adults, two-thirds of primary brain tumors are supratentorial; in children, two-thirds are infratentorial
- Gliomas, metastases, meningiomas, pituitary adenomas, and acoustic neuromas account for >95% of all brain tumors
- Clinically, present with epilepsy, raised intracranial pressure (ICP), or focal neurological deficits

HARDCORE

Glioblastoma multiforme (GM) is the most common and most aggressive primary brain tumor; seen in older (45–70 years) individuals. High-grade astrocytic tumor that is often rapidly fatal. Although any brain region can be affected, most commonly found in frontal and temporal lobes, as well as the basal ganglia. Transcallosal spread ("butterfly glioma") common. Classic histologic finding of "*pseudopalisading necrosis*."

HARDCORE

Meningiomas may arise from any part of the meninges from the falx, or from the tentorium. Second most common primary intracranial brain tumor and most common nonglial tumor; nearly always benign. Supratentorial, frequenting the parasagittal dural convexities. Majority are asymptomatic and solitary, but up to 10% are multiple and associated with *neurofibromatosis type II*. Pathology shows characteristic concentric *whorls* and calcified *psammoma bodies*.

HARDCORE

Pituitary adenomas are the most common tumors of pituitary gland. May be supra- or parasellar. Produce two principal sets of symptoms: Visual field defects (classic *bitemporal hemianopsia* from compression of optic chiasm) and endocrine disturbance (*prolactinoma* most common). *Pituitary apoplexy* (acute hypopituitarism) occurs secondary to acute infarction (e.g., Sheehan's syndrome).

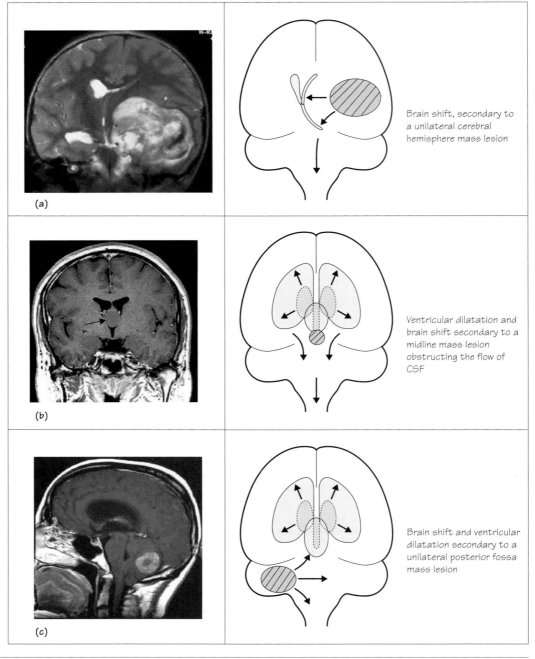

HARDCORE

Signs and symptoms manifesting acute increases in intracranial pressure depend on location of mass. Presence of mass lesions results in *transtentorial herniation and medullary coning*. A unilateral cerebral hemisphere mass shifts brain structures laterally and inferomedially (**a**), causing decreased consciousness (reticular activating system), respiratory depression (medulla), and pupil dilatation (CN 3). *Ventricular dilatation* and brain shift occur secondary to a midline mass lesion that obstructs downward flow of CSF (**b**). A mass in the posterior fossa (**c**) may result in compression of the fourth ventricle (ventricular dilatation) and *tonsillar herniation*.

Brain shift, secondary to a unilateral cerebral hemisphere mass lesion

Ventricular dilatation and brain shift secondary to a midline mass lesion obstructing the flow of CSF

Brain shift and ventricular dilatation secondary to a unilateral posterior fossa mass lesion

Figure 14-2 Consequences of acute increased ICP depend on site of lesion, and include brain shifts, herniation, and ventricular dilatation (**a, b, c**). (Reprinted with permission from Wilkinson I. Essential Neurology. 4th ed. Oxford: Blackwell Publishing, 2005:43.)

Brain Tumors More Commonly Found in Children

In children, CNS tumors are second in incidence only to leukemias.

Astrocytoma

- Account for majority of children's brain tumors
- Most are low-grade, cystic, slow-growing, and localized
- Typically histology include "Rosenthal fibers" and "pilocytic astrocytes"
- Surgery can be curative

Medulloblastoma

- Most common malignant brain tumor in children
- Most often arises in posterior fossa (in the fourth ventricle, between brainstem and cerebellum)
- Primitive neuroectodermal tumor (**PNET**)
- Invasive, frequently metastasize via CSF
- Highly radiosensitive

Ependymoma

- Almost always benign, but can obstruct flow of CSF
- Arises from ependymal lining of ventricle (usually fourth); in adults, occur most commonly in spinal cord
- Up to 70% found in posterior fossa

Other Tumors and Cysts

- Craniopharyngiomas (remnants of Rathke's pouch, bitemporal hemianopsia, hypopituitarism, calcification)
- Colloid cysts (third ventricle remnant, acute obstructive hydrocephalous)
- Hemangioblastoma (vascular, mostly cerebellum, von Hippel-Lindau syndrome)

INTRACRANIAL BLEEDS

Epidural Hematoma

- Traumatic accumulation of blood in epidural space caused by focused blow to head
- Tearing of *middle meningeal artery*; overlying fracture common
- Fibrous dura separates slowly
- Classic "*football*" or "*lens-shaped*" mass on CT that does not cross suture lines
- *Lucid interval* often follows initial loss of consciousness
- Increasing headache and drowsiness (mass effect) signal expansion of bleed requiring surgical decompression

Subdural Hematoma

- Formed by bleeding of cerebral *bridging veins* penetrating meninges; may be acute, subacute, or chronic
- Arachnoid and dura come apart easily
- Most common in elderly patients, especially with *alcohol abuse*
- "*Crescentic*" feature on CT that crosses suture lines
- Personality changes sometimes seen in chronic cases
- Consider child abuse if seen in young children

HARDCORE

Bleeding into the subarachnoid space is most commonly secondary to trauma, spontaneous *rupture of an aneurysm* (typically at junctions in the circle of Willis), and arteriovenous malformations (AVMs, often congenital). Patients with connective tissue disorders (e.g., Marfan's or Ehlers-Danlos syndrome) at higher risk for AVMs and aneurysms. Characteristics of *subarachnoid hemorrhage (SAH)* include sudden severe headaches (blood irritating meninges: "*Worst headache of my life*"), photophobia, and *meningismus*. Spasm of cerebral arteries can result in neurological deficits. Significant rebleeding risk without intervention (clipping of aneurysm). Small bleeds may not be detectable on CT, thus LP may be required to confirm diagnosis. CSF is *xanthochromic* because of presence of hemoglobin breakdown products.

CHAPTER 15

Hardcore Clinical Topics

In this section, a variety of clinical neurological problems are presented, with brief discussion of etiology, presentation, and management. Areas covered include myopathic disorders, disorders of equilibrium, dementia, and ischemic stroke.

MYOPATHIC DISORDERS

Muscular Dystrophies

Inherited muscle disorders characterized by progressive muscle weakness and wasting.

Duchenne's Dystrophy

- *Most common* form of muscular dystrophy
- *X-linked recessive disorder* affecting mostly males
- Results from deletion of *dystrophin gene*, leading to absent/reduced dystrophin protein in muscle
- Symptoms begin around *5 years of age*
- Early signs: Toe walking, waddling gait, inability to run
- Often see *Gowers' sign*: Using the arms to push off the legs in order to stand up
- *Pseudohypertrophy of calves* common (due to fatty infiltration of muscle)
- Distribution of muscle weakness: Pelvic, then shoulder girdle; eventually limb and respiratory muscles
- Creatine kinase levels high
- Steroids may improve muscle strength, but patients typically severely disabled by adolescence, with death in third decade
- Diagnosed by muscle biopsy and PCR

Becker's Dystrophy

- *X-linked recessive disorder*, with normal dystrophin levels, but alteration in protein
- Later onset and death than Duchenne's, but similar pattern of weakness (pelvic, then shoulder girdle)
- No cardiac or cognitive involvement

Congenital Myopathies

- Rare, relatively nonprogressive disorders that usually begin in infancy/childhood
- Characterized by proximal muscle weakness, hypotonia, hyporeflexia, normal serum creatine kinase; diagnosed by muscle biopsy

Nemaline Myopathy

- Characterized by *rod-shaped bodies* in muscle fibers

Central Core Disease

- Associated with *malignant hyperthermia*

Mitochondrial Myopathies

- Characterized by "*ragged red fibers*" that represent accumulations of abnormal mitochondria

KEARNS-SAYRE-DAROFF SYNDROME

- Progressive external ophthalmoplegia, retinal degeneration, cardiac conduction defects, cerebellar ataxia, elevated CSF protein

HARDCORE

Malignant hyperthermia:

- Autosomal dominant, results from defect on *ryanodine receptor* (calcium channel) gene
- Administration of *neuromuscular blocking agents* (e.g., succinylcholine) *or inhalational anesthetics* (e.g., halothane) results in rigidity, hyperthermia, metabolic acidosis, myoglobinuria
- 70% mortality
- Treatment: *Dantrolene* (ryanodine receptor antagonist), correction of acidosis, reduction of body temperature

HARDCORE

Vertigo (sense of movement of body or environment) and/or *ataxia* (incoordination of limbs or gait) are characteristic of equilibrium disorders. Vertigo can be either peripheral or central:

- *Peripheral vertigo:* Tends to be intermittent, always with nystagmus; commonly produces inner ear symptoms such as hearing loss/tinnitus
- *Central vertigo:* May have nystagmus; may see brainstem or cerebellar signs such as motor/sensory defects, hyperreflexia, Babinski's sign, dysarthria, or limb ataxia

MERRF

- Myoclonic epilepsy, ragged red fiber syndrome

MELAS

- Mitochondrial myopathy, encephalopathy, lactic acidosis, and strokelike episodes

Inflammatory Myopathies

Polymyositis/Dermatomyositis

- *Inflammatory infiltration* and destruction of muscle fibers
- Leads to *weakness/wasting*, especially in *proximal limb and girdle muscles*
- Dermatomyositis characterized by *heliotrope rash* (erythematous rash over eyelid or on extensor surfaces of joints) and Gottron's papules (erythematous papules/plaques over bony prominences)
- Associated with autoimmune disorders, positive anti-Jo 1 antibodies
- Dermatomyositis associated with malignancy
- Treatment: Steroids

AIDS-Associated Myopathies

- Polymyositis
- Type II muscle fiber atrophy
- Mitochondrial myopathy can result from antiretroviral treatment

DISORDERS OF EQUILIBRIUM

Along with the senses of touch and vision, the vestibular system is essential for maintaining balance.

Peripheral Vestibular Disorders

Benign Positional Vertigo

- Attacks of vertigo that occur in certain positions
- Etiologies include head trauma and canalolithiasis (debris floating in endolymph stimulates semicircular canal)

Ménière's Disease

- Repeated episodes of vertigo, progressive sensorineural hearing loss, and tinnitus
- Thought to result from idiopathic excess of endolymphatic fluid
- Some cases familial (related to mutations on *cochlin gene*)

Toxic Vestibulopathies

AMINOGLYCOSIDES

- Streptomycin, gentamicin, tobramycin most likely to cause *vestibular toxicity*
- Amikacin, kanamycin, tobramycin associated with *hearing loss*

SALICYLATES (ASPIRIN)

- Chronic and high-dose salicylates can cause reversible tinnitus, vertigo, and sensorineural hearing loss

QUININE AND QUINIDINE

- Can cause *cinchonism*
- Tinnitus, impaired hearing, vertigo, visual defects, nausea, vomiting, abdominal pain; severe cases can have fever, encephalopathy, coma, and death

Central Vestibular Disorders

Alcoholic Cerebellar Degeneration

- Progressive degeneration of *superior vermis* of cerebellum seen in *chronic alcoholics*; may include degeneration of *mammillary bodies*
- Most common in men from 40 to 60 years of age
- *Gait ataxia* universal feature

- Also can see sensory deficits in feet, ataxia of arms, nystagmus, dysarthria, hypotonia
- Likely results from nutritional deficiency of *vitamin B₁ (thiamine)*

Friedreich's Ataxia

- *Autosomal recessive* degenerative disorder due to GAA *trinucleotide repeat* in *frataxin gene* on chromosome 9
- Pathologic findings include degeneration of spinocerebellar tracts, posterior columns, dorsal roots
- Clinical manifestations usually occur *after 4 years of age* and include progressive gait ataxia, loss of knee and ankle tendon reflexes, cerebellar dysarthria; sensory abnormalities may develop, as well as kyphoscoliosis, cardiomyopathy, and visual impairment

Ataxia-Telangiectasia

- Autosomal recessive disorder resulting from *mutation in ATM gene*
- Onset of *pancerebellar degeneration in infancy*
- Patients develop mental deficiency and *oculocutaneous telangiectasias*
- Decreased levels of IgA result in increased respiratory infections
- Increased risk of malignancy (especially acute lymphocytic leukemia [ALL] and lymphoma)

DEMENTIA

Alzheimer's Disease

- Most common cause of dementia
- Usually sporadic, but 5% of cases have identifiable genetic basis
- High incidence in *trisomy 21* (Down's syndrome) patients
- Familial Alzheimer's disease is autosomal dominant, caused by a variety of known mutations
  - Mutation in *amyloid precursor protein* on Chromosome 21
  - Mutation in *presenilin 1* associated with especially early onset
  - Mutation in *presenilin 2* found in some families
- Additionally, risk of Alzheimer's associated with number of *apolipoprotein E4 alleles*

PATHOGENESIS

- Pathogenesis is unclear; however, Alzheimer's disease is defined by presence of *neuritic plaques* and *neurofibrillary tangles*
  - *Neuritic plaques*: Extracellular deposits principally composed of *β-amyloid*
    - β-amyloid normally results from cleavage of *amyloid precursor protein* (APP) and is cleared from brain; abnormal cleavage results in accumulation of β-amyloid in extracellular plaques
  - *Neurofibrillary tangles*: Intracellular deposits of *tau* (microtubule-associated protein) and ubiquitin
- Cholinergic neurons are lost, and acetylcholine-synthesizing enzyme is markedly reduced in cerebral cortex and hippocampus

CLINICAL MANIFESTATIONS

- Impairment of *recent memory* progressing to disorientation to time, place, then person
- Patients eventually develop aphasia, anomia, apraxia, and psychiatric symptoms
- Death occurs 5–10 years after onset of symptoms

TREATMENT

- *Cholinesterase inhibitors* to balance relative deficiency of cholinergic signaling
  - Donepezil, rivastigmine
- No drugs are known to alter disease progression

Pick's Disease

- Distinguished from Alzheimer's disease by histological appearance at autopsy and *younger age of onset* (40–60)
- Histology shows *swollen/ballooned neurons (Pick cells)* and *neuronal inclusions* on *silver staining (Pick bodies)*

HARDCORE

Some potentially reversible causes of dementia:

- Depression (pseudodementia)
- Metabolic disorders
- Normal pressure hydrocephalus
- Intracranial mass lesions
- Vitamin B₁₂ deficiency
- Hypothyroidism
- Neurosyphilis
- Drug intoxication

Prion proteins exist in normal neurons; abnormal prions *induce a conformational change* in normal prions and result in *prion disease.*

- Human diseases caused by prions include:
  - Creutzfeld-Jakob disease (sporadic and familial)
  - Kuru (thought to be spread by cannibalism in New Guinea)
  - Fatal familial insomnia
- Animal diseases caused by prions include:
  - Bovine spongiform encephalopathy ("mad cow disease")

The *sudden loss of function* is a hallmark sign of cerebrovascular disease (stroke). This typically occurs via one of two etiologies:

- *Ischemia/infarction*
  - Caused by occlusion of arteries supplying brain
  - Common cause of stroke resulting in wide range of outcomes
- *Hemorrhage*
  - Intracranial bleeding as the result of trauma or spontaneous rupture of vessel
  - Less common than ischemic stroke, and typically causes higher morbidity/ mortality

Atheroma formation in the carotid artery can result in small emboli traveling to the retinal artery, causing blockages and *transient monocular blindness*, a condition termed *amaurosis fugax*. Patients may say that "a curtain comes down" over their eye. Such symptoms are indicative of vascular disease and increased risk for stroke. Workup includes *carotid ultrasound*. If artery is blocked > 70%, patient may be candidate for surgical removal of atheroma (carotid endarterectomy) or stenting to reduce risk of stroke.

Occlusion of a cerebral artery results in ischemia to the region of the brain supplied by that artery and loss of function controlled by the affected area. When the embolic material is lysed/fragmented before permanent damage has ensued, the patient may regain neurological function of that tissue.

- When symptoms resolve *within 24 hours and there is no detectable infarct on imaging*, the patient is said to have had a transient ischemic attack (TIA)
  - *One-third of patients with TIAs will have a stroke within 5 years*
- Complete resolution of symptoms in more than 24 hours is termed a reversible ischemic neurological deficit (RIND)

- Neurodegeneration initially confined to frontal and temporal lobes
- Presents with *frontal dementia*; changes in personality, social behavior, higher executive function

Vascular Dementia

- Dementia thought to result from multiple infarcts secondary to cerebrovascular disease
- Second most common cause of dementia after Alzheimer's disease
- Patients typically have history of hypertension, stepwise progression of deficits, and either multiple large cortical infarcts or many smaller infarcts
- Subcortical white matter, basal ganglia, or thalamus typically affected on MRI
- Rule out other causes of multiple infarcts: Cardiac emboli, cerebral vasculitis, polycythemia, meningovascular syphilis

AIDS Dementia Complex

- *Most common neurologic manifestation of AIDS*
- HIV infects monocytes, macrophages, and microglia of CNS
- Unclear pathogenesis, but such infection can result in cognitive and behavioral symptoms
- Symptoms progress with time, and include memory loss, dementia, ataxia, hyperreflexia, among other changes

Progressive Multifocal Leukoencephalopathy

- Progressive dementia and cortical dysfunction (hemiparesis, visual deficits, aphasia, sensory impairment) resulting from infection with or reactivation of latent *JC virus* (a papovavirus)
- Most common in *immunosuppressed patients*
- Infection of oligodendrocytes causes patchy *demyelination* of white matter of cerebral hemispheres, as well as brainstem and cerebellum
- Death occurs in 3–6 months

Creutzfeldt-Jakob Disease

- Fatal transmissible disorder caused by abnormal *prions*
- Patients develop *progressive dementia*, psychiatric symptoms, startle myoclonus, extrapyramidal signs
- Pathology includes spongiform changes in brain, neuronal loss, and gliosis
- Death usually occurs within 1 year

CEREBROVASCULAR DISEASE

Ischemic Stroke

- Caused by *occlusion of vessel* by local thrombus formation or embolic material delivered from another vessel or the heart
- Common conditions resulting in ischemia and subsequent infarction:
  - *Cardiac disease* associated with embolization (e.g., atrial fibrillation, mural thrombus following myocardial infarction, valvular disease, endocarditis)
  - *Atheroma* of large neck arteries (associated signs and symptoms include previous myocardial infarction, angina pectoris, intermittent leg claudication)
  - *Hematologic disorders* (e.g., polycythemia, sickle cell disease, hypercoagulable states)

RISK FACTORS

- Same risk factors for coronary artery disease
  - *Hypertension*
  - *Diabetes*
  - *Hyperlipidemia*
  - *Smoking*
  - *Obesity*

CLINICAL PRESENTATION

- Depends on artery involved and territory supplied
- Neurological deficits can often be localized to an area supplied by either the anterior or posterior circulation

TABLE 15–1 Anterior Cerebral Circulation

VESSEL	AREA SUPPLIED	ASSOCIATED DEFICIT
Ophthalmic artery (arises from internal carotid artery)	Retina	Transient monocular blindness (amaurosis fugax)
Middle cerebral artery (MCA) and lenticulostriate branches *Because the MCA is the largest branch of the carotid, it is the most common artery involved in ischemic stroke*	• Motor and sensory representation of face, hand, arm • Expressive and receptive language areas • Basal ganglia and motor fibers of face, hand, arm, and leg as they pass through internal capsule	• Contralateral hemiparesis and hemisensory deficit of face, hand, and arm, sparing the leg (unless lenticulostriates are involved) • Broca's or Wernicke's aphasia if dominant hemisphere involved • Homonymous hemianopsia • Neglect, apraxia
Anterior cerebral artery	• Motor and sensory representation of leg (parasagittal cerebral cortex) • Bladder inhibitory center	• Contralateral paralysis and sensory loss of leg • Loss of voluntary control of micturition

TABLE 15–2 Posterior Cerebral Circulation

VESSEL	AREA SUPPLIED	ASSOCIATED DEFICIT
Posterior cerebral artery	• Occipital cerebral cortex • Medial temporal lobes • Thalamus • Rostral midbrain	• Contralateral homonymous hemianopsia (possibly sparing macular vision because of dual supply to this region by MCA) • Difficulty naming, reading, identifying objects • Cortical blindness
Basilar artery	• Occipital and temporal lobes • Thalamus • Internal capsule • Brainstem and cerebellum	• Hemiplegia or quadriplegia • Coma • "Locked-in" syndrome
Branches of vertebral and basilar arteries: • Posterior inferior cerebellar artery (PICA) • Anterior inferior cerebellar artery (AICA)	• Dorsolateral brainstem and associated cranial nerves • Cerebellar peduncles	Occlusion of PICA results in Wallenberg's syndrome: vertigo, nausea, vomiting, dysphagia, hoarseness, nystagmus, ipsilateral Horner's syndrome, limb ataxia
Lacunar vessels (lenticulostriate arteries deep in brain)	• Putamen, thalamus, pons, internal capsule	• Pure motor hemiparesis • Pure sensory stroke • Mixed motor/sensory deficits

HARDCORE

Areas for *receptive and expressive language* are located around the *lateral (Sylvian) sulcus of the dominant hemisphere* in the majority of people (e.g., in a right-handed person, language areas are found in the left hemisphere). *Global aphasia*: All language areas are damaged, with resulting loss of comprehension, fluent speech, and repetition.

HARDCORE

Wernicke's area:
• Responsible for *receptive* language
• A lesion here results in Wernicke's aphasia, in which the patient *cannot comprehend* language, but can still produce fluent, although usually nonsensical speech
• Remember: *Wernicke's* aphasia is "*wordy*"

HARDCORE

Broca's Area
• Responsible for *expressive* language
• A lesion here results in Broca's aphasia, in which *patients comprehend*, but cannot speak fluently; they may stutter, or be unable to name objects
• Remember: Speech in *Broca's* aphasia is "*broken*"

HARDCORE

Wernicke's and Broca's areas are connected by the *arcuate fasciculus*.
• A lesion here produces conductive aphasia: Patients comprehend and can speak, but *cannot repeat*

Stroke Management

TRANSIENT ISCHEMIC ATTACK (TIA)

• TIA of *noncardiogenic* etiology (e.g., atherosclerosis/thrombosis)
  ○ Treatment: Antiplatelet therapy
• TIA of *cardiac* etiology (e.g., atrial fibrillation, patent foramen ovale, endocarditis)
  ○ Treatment: Anticoagulation with heparin/warfarin
    – Risk of anticoagulant therapy includes intracranial hemorrhage (greatest in patients > 65 and those with hypertension)
  ○ Other treatments: Carotid endarterectomy, angioplasty, and stenting

COMPLETED ISCHEMIC STROKE

• Treatment: Intravenous thrombolytic therapy (must rule out hemorrhagic stroke first)
• *Recombinant tissue plasminogen activator (r-tPA)*
  ○ Serine protease that lyses fibrin-containing clots
  ○ Must be given *within 3 hours of onset* of symptoms
  Cannot be given if patient has been anticoagulated, has recently bled, or if diagnosis uncertain (because of risk of hemorrhage)

CHAPTER 16

Hardcore Imaging

Despite the importance of an accurate history and a sound physical exam in neurological diagnoses, it is often necessary to apply special investigative technologies to patients in order to arrive at a definitive diagnosis or to provide objective evidence for one's clinical suspicions. Noninvasive imaging techniques (such as CT and MRI) have revolutionized the diagnosis of neurology patients. Know the major findings on CT/MRI for some of the most often tested diseases, as well as their indications and contraindications. Most of what appears on the USMLE will be obvious.

PLAIN X-RAYS

Simple, plain x-rays of the skull, facial bones, and spine have now fallen out of favor and have *limited usefulness beyond settings of acute trauma* (when a fracture is suspected).

- Plain x-rays of the cervical spine can demonstrate abnormalities of the vertebrae, narrowing of disc spaces, and osteophytic projections in the intervetebral foramina
- Lumbar x-rays are less informative but can demonstrate disc degeneration or spondylolisthesis

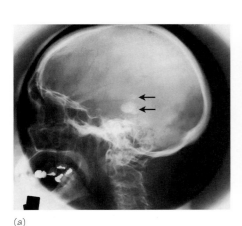

(a)

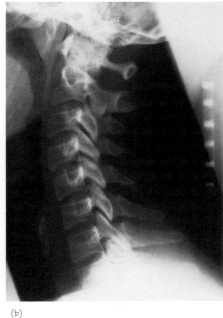

(b)

Figure 16-1 Normal lateral plain x-rays of a skull (a) and cervical spine (b). Prominent calcifications (arrows in a) denote the pineal gland and choroid plexus. (Reprinted with permission from Ginsberg L. Lecture Notes: Neurology. 8th ed. Oxford: Blackwell Publishing, 2005:54.)

COMPUTERIZED AXIAL TOMOGRAPHY

Computerized axial tomography (CAT) scan, more commonly known as CT scan, uses special x-rays and computers to capture *cross-sectional images of body tissues and organs*. CT has revolutionized the investigation of neurological disease states (e.g., intracranial lesions) as well as spinal processes. Its main advantage is speed, especially for detection of acute hemorrhages. Images can be refined further with administration of IV contrast medium to highlight areas of increased vascularity, regions of blood-brain barrier breakdown, aneurysms, or arteriovenous malformations.

HARDCORE

Abnormalities detectable on head CT:
- Presence of blood (hemorrhages) and bone (both seen better than with MRI)
- Calcium/calcifications
- Most strokes/infarcts
- Tumors and other intracranial lesions
- Hydrocephalus
- Cerebral atrophy/edema
- Check for *mass effect* from any lesion seen on head CT, evidenced by compression of ventricles or midline structure shifts

MAGNETIC RESONANCE IMAGING

Magnetic resonance imaging (MRI) depends on the response of the body's hydrogen ions to a strong magnetic field and provides information on the physical properties of the tissue (e.g., water content). MRI does not require x-rays. Two types of "weighted imaging" are based on spinning and relaxation states of protons—T1-weighted images show *changes in tissue homogeneity* (tumors, dead tissue), while T2-weighted images are useful to demonstrate an *increase in fluid content* (vasogenic or cytotoxic edema). For instance, CSF appears dark on T1-weighted images (while fat and soft tissue appear bright) and very bright on T2-weighted images.

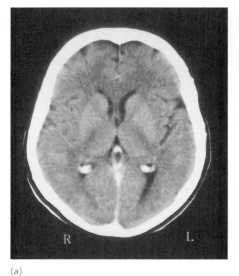

(a)

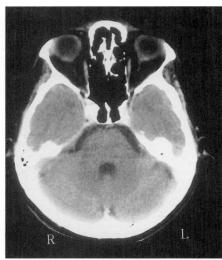

(b)

Figure 16-2 Normal head CT scans showing the cerebral hemispheres (a) and the temporal lobes and posterior fossa (b). The bony structures have a white-out appearance. (Reprinted with permission from Ginsberg L. Lecture Notes: Neurology. 8th ed. Oxford: Blackwell Publishing, 2005:54.)

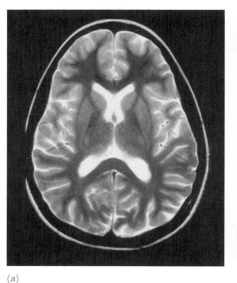

(a)

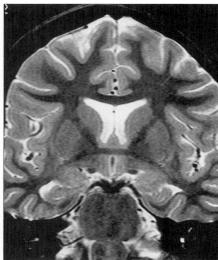

(b)

Figure 16-3 Normal MRI scans of the brain, showing the axial (a) and coronal (b) sections. Major structures seen in gross anatomy can be clearly differentiated. White matter tracts appear white. Anteroposterior view of neck vessels from MRA (c). (Reprinted with permission from Ginsberg L. Lecture Notes: Neurology. 8th ed. Oxford: Blackwell Publishing, 2005:55–56.)

(c)

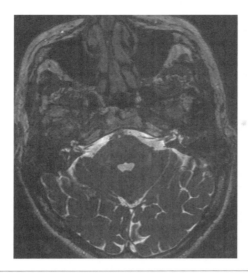

Figure 16-4 Normal MRI of the head with T2-weighting (CSF is bright in this image). (Courtesy of Cedars-Sinai Medical Center, Los Angeles, California.)

- Provides better resolution than is possible with CT
- Images can be reconstructed in any plane (sagittal, coronal, axial)
- Great for diseases of the posterior cranial fossa, gray and white matters
- Ideal for spinal column, cord, and nerve roots
- MR angiography (MRA) images blood vessels (gadolinium as contrast)
- Less sensitive than CT in evaluating calcifications and subtle fractures
- *Contraindications* include cardiac pacemaker, metallic foreign bodies

ANGIOGRAPHY

Injection of a contrast medium into the circulation, usually by means of a catheter inserted into the femoral artery and threaded up the vascular tree, demonstrates the carotid or vertebrobasilar vessels. A series of x-rays is then taken to follow flow.

- Ideal for *aneurysms, angiomas, blood supplies to tumors*
- Small risks of ischemia from embolism, hypotension, or vasospasm
- Interventional techniques employed to coil, embolize, and stent vascular lesions

HARDCORE

Abnormalities detectable on brain MRI:
- CNS infections (abscesses)
- Noninfectious inflammatory disease (e.g., multiple sclerosis)
- Evaluation of stroke acutely (via perfusion and diffusion imaging)
- Pre-/postoperative or treatment evaluation of brain tumors
- Meningeal disease

HARDCORE

Abnormalities detectable on spinal MRI:
- Infection/inflammatory disease
- Primary tumors/metastases
- Initial evaluation of syrinx
- Evaluation of disk herniation versus scarring

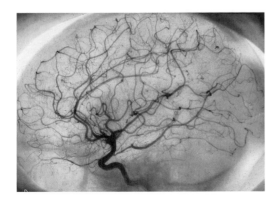

Figure 16-5 Normal internal carotid arteriogram (via angiography). (Reprinted with permission from Ginsberg L. Lecture Notes: Neurology. 8th ed. Oxford: Blackwell Publishing, 2005:56.)

IMAGES

The following are images of normal anatomy and common neurologic disorders.

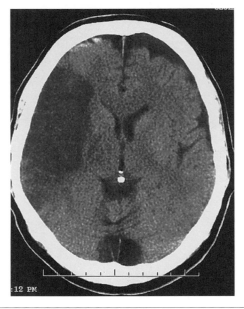

Figure 16-6 Head CT of a cerebral infarction, involving the right MCA. CT may not be required in every patient (particularly if clinical diagnosis is clear-cut), but is useful to distinguish between cerebral infarction and hemorrhage. Also eliminates important differential diagnoses (tumor, infection, hematoma). (Reprinted with permission from Ginsberg L. Lecture Notes: Neurology. 8th ed. Oxford: Blackwell Publishing, 2005:83.)

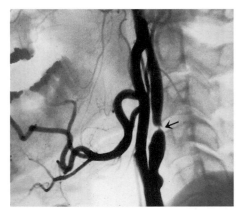

Figure 16-7 Angiography demonstrating severe stenosis of the internal carotid artery (arrow). Used to detect carotid stenosis in patients with TIAs in the carotid territory. (Reprinted with permission from Ginsberg L. Lecture Notes: Neurology. 8th ed. Oxford: Blackwell Publishing, 2005:86.)

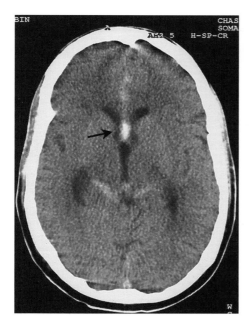

Figure 16-8 Head CT of a subarachnoid hemorrhage. Regions of high density, representing blood, are widespread but particularly evident in the interhemispheric fissure (arrow). This patient had bled from an anterior communicating artery aneurysm. (Reprinted with permission from Ginsberg L. Lecture Notes: Neurology. 8th ed. Oxford: Blackwell Publishing, 2005:88.)

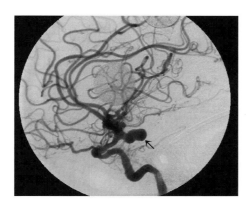

Figure 16-9 Carotid angiogram showing a posterior communicating artery aneurysm (arrow). (Reprinted with permission from Ginsberg L. Lecture Notes: Neurology. 8th ed. Oxford: Blackwell Publishing, 2005:88.)

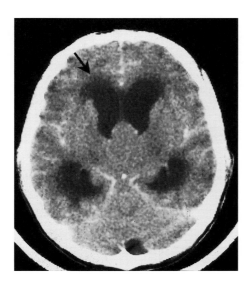

Figure 16-10 Head CT of an obstructive hydrocephalus. The arrow points to the periventricular lucency (low density) that is indicative of cerebral edema. Dilated lateral ventricles, as well as a mass at the level of the third ventricle that is presumably responsible for blocking CSF outflow can be appreciated. (Reprinted with permission from Ginsberg L. Lecture Notes: Neurology. 8th ed. Oxford: Blackwell Publishing, 2005:104.)

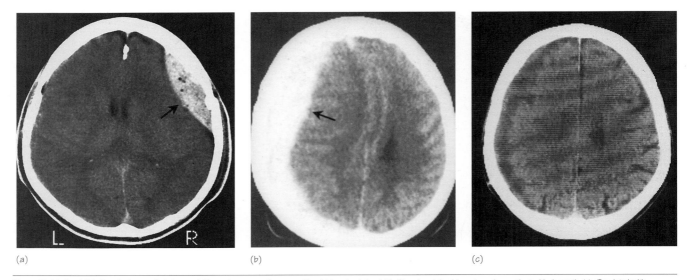

(a)   (b)   (c)

Figure 16-11 Head CT of acute traumatic intracranial hematomas—extra- or epidural (a) and subdural (b). Chronic subdural hematoma in a patient with dementia (**c**). (Reprinted with permission from Ginsberg L. Lecture Notes: Neurology. 8th ed. Oxford: Blackwell Publishing, 2005:106,157.)

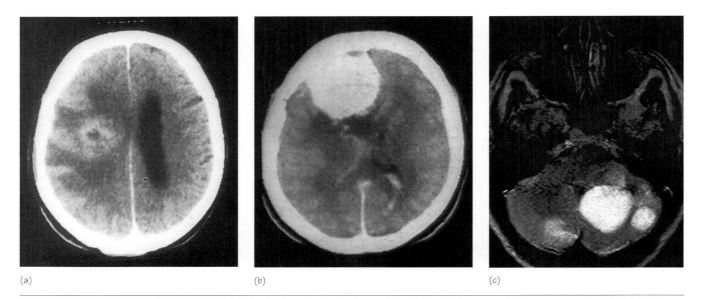

(a)   (b)   (c)

Figure 16-12 Head CT of a cerebral glioma that has invaded the right lateral ventricle (**a**) and **an intracranial meningioma (b)** that has caused shifting of structures (mass effect). Axial MRI showing **cerebellar metastases (c)**. Metastatic cancer commonly involves the brain, particular in the case of primary lung, breast, and bowel tumors. (Reprinted with permission from Ginsberg L. Lecture Notes: Neurology. 8th ed. Oxford: Blackwell Publishing, 2005:107–108,167.)

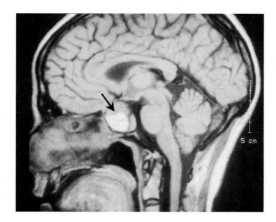

Figure 16-13 Sagittal MRI of the brain showing presence of a pituitary adenoma (arrow). The increased high signal within the pituitary is secondary to hemorrhage within the tumor. (Reprinted with permission from Ginsberg L. Lecture Notes: Neurology. 8th ed. Oxford: Blackwell Publishing, 2005:108.)

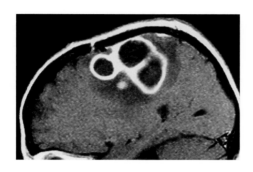

Figure 16-14 Parasagittal brain MRI demonstrating a multilocular cerebral abscess. The prominent high-signal "ring enhancements" are secondary to infusion of gadolinium contrast. The surrounding edema can be appreciated as low-intensity signals around the lesion. (Reprinted with permission from Ginsberg L. Lecture Notes: Neurology. 8th ed. Oxford: Blackwell Publishing, 2005:113.)

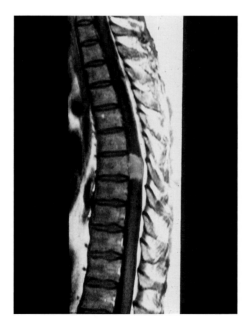

Figure 16-15 Sagittal MRI of the thoracic spine showing a spinal meningioma, causing cord compression. A timely diagnosis is essential to maximizing chances of a successful surgical intervention. (Reprinted with permission from Ginsberg L. Lecture Notes: Neurology. 8th ed. Oxford: Blackwell Publishing, 2005:124.)

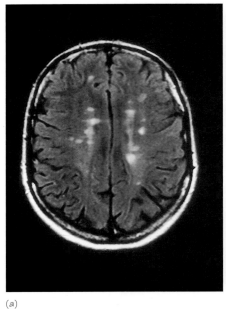

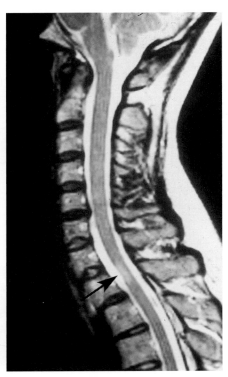

Figure 16-16 MRI of brain in multiple sclerosis.
White areas (**a**) represent multiple lesions in both
hemispheres, with the typical periventricular
demyelination pattern. The plaques can also be seen
elsewhere, as evidenced by focal cord atrophy (arrow) at
the level of the cervical spinal cord (**b**). (Reprinted with
permission from Ginsberg L. Lecture Notes: Neurology.
8th ed. Oxford: Blackwell Publishing, 2005:133.)

(a)

(b)

CHAPTER 17

Step 1 Practice Questions and Answers

1. An 18-year-old woman falls while rollerblading and strikes the left side of her head against a concrete wall at the park. On physical examination, only a minor scalp abrasion is present at the site of the impact, with minimal bleeding that had stopped after a few minutes. She is initially alert following this accident, but then becomes unconscious 20 minutes later. A stat head CT scan reveals a convex, lens-shaped area of hemorrhage centered over the left parietal region. Which of the following is the most likely intracranial structure to have been damaged?
   A. Middle cerebral artery
   B. Cavernous sinus
   C. Great vein of Galen
   D. Middle meningeal artery
   E. Inferior cerebellar artery
   F. Maxillary branch of external carotid artery

2. You are asked to see a 61-year-old Asian man who has been placed in an assisted-living facility by his daughters because he can no longer be cared for at home. He has had increasing difficulty keeping his room in order. He misplaces articles of clothing, is unable to appropriately dress himself, and has become increasingly incontinent over the last few months. These problems have gotten progressively worse over the past 5 years, such that he has been found wandering aimlessly around the neighborhood on several occasions. His family tells you that he had taken early retirement as a college math teacher because he was having trouble grading his exams and executing his lesson plans. They deny any history of trauma or seizures. Which specific cellular findings would one expect to encounter as being most representative of his underlying disease process?
   A. Muscle atrophy with loss of anterior horn cells
   B. Atrophy of caudate nuclei
   C. Neurofibrillary tangles and neuritic plaques
   D. Depigmentation of the substantia nigra
   E. Nonspecific Wallerian degeneration

3. As the third-year medical student on the neurology ward team, you are asked by your attending to test an elderly woman's palatal movements. When she is asked to say "ah," you observe that the left side of her palate is at a lower level than her right and that her uvula is deviated toward the right. You tell your team that this patient most likely has suffered a lesion to her:
   A. Left glossopharyngeal nerve
   B. Right glossopharyngeal nerve
   C. Left vagus nerve
   D. Right vagus nerve
   E. Left spinal accessory nerve
   F. Right spinal accessory nerve

4. A previously healthy 33-year-old man presents to the ER with a 2-hour history of a severe headache, photophobia, nausea, and vomiting, and promptly loses consciousness as you are about to take a more detailed history. A stat head CT scan reveals extensive hemorrhage at the base of the brain. He is afebrile, bradycardic, and hypertensive. You detect papilledema on funduscopic exam. Lumbar puncture (LP) yields CSF with frank blood that fails to clear, no white blood cells (WBCs), normal glucose, and slightly elevated protein levels. What is the most likely diagnosis?
   A. Creutzfeldt-Jakob disease
   B. Ruptured berry aneurysm
   C. Progressive multifocal leukoencephalopathy (PML)
   D. Huntington's disease
   E. Acute bacterial meningitis

5. A 65-year-old African American man has had transient ischemic attacks (TIAs) for the past 2 years. He presents to your clinic complaining of diplopia, ataxia, and vertigo. Upon further questioning he admits to also having had episodes of sudden bilateral visual loss in the past few months. Which of the following underlying conditions can you safely place near the bottom of your differential?
   A. Coronary atherosclerosis
   B. Cerebellar tumor
   C. Cholesterol emboli on funduscopic exam
   D. Stenosis of proximal subclavian artery on angiography
   E. Cardiac arrhythmias

6. A 52-year-old woman has had symptoms of dementia with marked frontal lobe features of grandiosity and antisocial behavior for the past 4 years. On physical examination, she walks with an ataxic stamping gait; knee and ankle reflexes are absent. Laboratory studies from both blood and CSF show VDRL positivity. In addition, the CSF protein and glucose are slightly elevated, and there are 25 lymphocytes per microliter. Which of the following pathologic findings is most likely to be present in her spinal cord?
   A. Loss of anterior horn cells
   B. Plaques of demyelination
   C. Atrophy of dorsal columns
   D. Diffuse hemorrhages
   E. Spondylotic myelopathy

7. Several members of a large multigenerational family (one of whom is your patient) are affected by progressive dementia and chorea, with an average age of onset of 35–40 years. The disorder appears to be autosomal dominant with trinucleotide CAG repeats by DNA analysis. The condition is relentless and death ensues usually within 15 years. Which of the following structures is most likely to be grossly abnormal (in addition to generalized cerebral atrophy) at autopsy of these patients?
   A. Caudate nucleus
   B. Cerebellum
   C. Frontal and temporal lobes
   D. Locus ceruleus
   E. Corticospinal tract

8. A 76-year-old woman was brought to the memory clinic because her family had noted worsening selective amnesia (particularly for recent events) for the past 11 months, with a tendency to confabulation. She dies 6 months from complications secondary to a hepatocellular carcinoma. At autopsy, microhemorrhages are visible in the brainstem and diencephala, as well as bilateral small mammillary bodies with brown discoloration. Which of the following is the most likely diagnosis?
   A. Chronic subdural hematoma
   B. Diffuse cortical Lewy body disease
   C. Wernicke-Korsakoff syndrome
   D. Alzheimer's disease
   E. Huntington's disease

9. A 35-year-old man had been recovering from a recent upper respiratory tract infection when he noticed weakness in both legs while walking up the stairs in his apartment. The weakness did not improve with rest. He had also developed numbness over parts of his lower extremities. The next day, while shaving in the shower, he noticed sudden weakness of the muscles on the right side of his face. On exam, the patient was not in apparent distress and was afebrile. Motor exam revealed obvious muscle weakness bilaterally, especially below his knees. Lower extremity deep tendon reflexes were markedly diminished. Sensory exam of the legs was significant for decreased pain and touch sensations in a stocking distribution; you also note a mild facial nerve palsy on the right side of his face. What is the most likely diagnosis?
   A. Myasthenia gravis
   B. Diabetic neuropathy
   C. Polyradiculopathy
   D. Guillain-Barré syndrome
   E. Amyotrophic lateral sclerosis

10. A 38-year-old woman presents to your office with an insidious onset of progressive weakness and dysphagia over the last 3 months. She has had difficulty walking up stairs at her home and has been experiencing difficulty swallowing solids. She denies having any numbness of her extremities, muscle tenderness, joint pains, incontinence, diarrhea, diplopia, weight loss,

or new rashes. Your exam revealed weakness of neck flexion with good neck extension. Extraocular movements were intact, facial strength was normal, and there was no ptosis and orbicularis oculi. Motor examination showed weakness of biceps, triceps, arm abductors, hip flexors, and quadriceps; sensory testing was within normal limits. Deep tendon reflexes were 2+ bilaterally. Cerebellar testing revealed dysmetria in proportion to her weakness. There was no evidence of joint tenderness or swelling. What is your diagnosis?
- A. Systemic lupus erythematosus (SLE) myopathy
- B. Toxoplasmosis
- C. Dermatomyositis
- D. Hyperthyroidism
- E. Lambert-Eaton syndrome
- F. Polymyositis

11. A 41-year-old man noticed tinnitus in his right ear that has progressed over the last 4 weeks to worsening hearing loss. On exam, he has decreased hearing on the left, with air conduction better than bone conduction. The rest of his cranial nerves are grossly intact. An MRI of his brain showed a discrete 2.5-cm mass located at the right cerebellopontine angle. What is the most appropriate statement to tell your patient?
- A. He probably has lesions elsewhere in his body
- B. Other members of his family should be screened for the same condition
- C. This is a benign tumor and he should do well after surgical resection
- D. He is likely to be HIV-positive
- E. The disease is likely to be chronic with remissions and exacerbations

12. A 40-year-old HIV-positive homeless woman is brought to the ER by her companion because of episodes of headaches over the past 2 months. Her companion denies a history of seizures, fever, chills, rashes, weight loss, anorexia, shortness of breath, or changes in bowel or urinary habits. On examination she has difficulty speaking full sentences. She is unable to follow simple commands or perform simple calculations and appears to perseverate. Multiple, bilateral, irregular ring-enhancing lesions in the white matter of her frontal lobe are found on MRI. Her current CD4 count is 115 per microliter. Which of the following is the most appropriate treatment option?
- A. Long course of IV broad-spectrum antibiotics
- B. Aggressive anti-HIV regimen
- C. High-dose chemotherapy and radiation
- D. Pyrimethamine, folinic acid, and clindamycin
- E. Nothing needs to be done—follow her condition with serial scans

13. A 42-year-old homeless woman is brought to the emergency department by her companion, who tells you that she has been vomiting and alternating between a lethargic and an agitated state for the last few days. The companion also describes her as being disoriented with disorganized thinking and altered sleep patterns. On admission, she is afebrile, with blood pressure of 120/80 mm Hg, pulse 75 per minute, and respirations 20 per minute. Her labs reveal a serum sodium of 115 mmol/L, potassium 4.0 mmol/L, and chloride 90 mmol/L. IV fluid is administered, and the serum sodium increases to 140 mmol/L the next morning. The patient's mental status improves, she becomes more alert, but deteriorates 24 hours later and dies. What do you expect to find at autopsy?
- A. Multiple watershed infarctions
- B. Periventricular plaques of demyelination
- C. Central pontine myelinolysis
- D. Intraparenchymal brain hemorrhage
- E. Widespread spongiform encephalopathy
- F. Subarachnoid hemorrhage

14. A mother brings her 5-year-old son to the pediatrician, concerned that he has started tip-toeing frequently and no longer runs. On exam, the pediatrician notices that the child has disproportionately large calves, and seems to push off his thighs to get up from a seated position. What protein is associated with this child's disorder?
- A. Actin
- B. Myosin
- C. Dystrophin
- D. Kinesin
- E. Troponin

15. A 61-year-old diabetic woman collapsed while walking her dog and was taken to the emergency room. After recovering consciousness, she is found to have right-sided weakness and

sensory loss, mostly involving her leg. She is able to speak normally, and has no difficulty swallowing. Given this presentation, occlusion of which artery likely led to her presentation?
A. Right middle cerebral
B. Left middle cerebral
C. Right anterior cerebral
D. Left anterior cerebral
E. Basilar

16. A 32-year-old white woman comes to your clinic complaining of double vision. She also reports difficulty balancing and occasional urinary incontinence. CT demonstrates diffuse lesions involving the brain and spinal cord. With which HLA haplotype is her disease associated?
A. DR2
B. DR3
C. DR4
D. B27
E. A3

17. One of your patients confides that she thinks her husband might have had a stroke. She notices that his head droops, and he seems to have difficulty talking and swallowing. Her husband is a 68-year-old man with a 30 pack-year smoking history. On questioning, he states that he does notice more weakness than before, particularly when trying to lift heavy objects, but says that after a few tries, his muscles "warm up," and he's fine. After examining him, you tell his wife that you don't think he has had a stroke. However, his collection of symptoms are of concern for what underlying process?
A. Multiple sclerosis
B. Small cell carcinoma of the lung
C. Brain tumor
D. Renal failure
E. Myasthenia gravis

18. A 30-year-old field worker is brought to the emergency room having difficulty breathing. He is sweating profusely, salivating, and his eyes are watering. His friend reports that the patient's illness started with diarrhea that afternoon. What do you suspect is going on with this patient?
A. Food poisoning
B. Organophosphate poisoning
C. Amphetamine overdose
D. Asthma exacerbation
E. Poisonous mushroom ingestion

19. During your pediatrics rotation, you see a 12-year-old girl who spent the previous weekend camping in the woods of Connecticut with her family. She came to the doctor's office because she now has a fever with chills, headache, and muscle aches. Upon further questioning, she recalls seeing a reddish rash with a clear center on her thigh. What cranial nerve is most often affected in this condition?
A. 3 (oculomotor)
B. 7 (facial)
C. 9 (glossopharyngeal)
D. 10 (vagus)
E. 12 (hypoglossal)

20. A 32-year-old man was brought to the hospital by ambulance after having a seizure. His wife reported that he had a fever and had complained of a headache. Lumbar puncture yielded CSF with elevated lymphocytes and protein. Intravenous treatment with the appropriate agent was begun, and the patient seemed to recover over several days. During his recovery, however, his wife noticed that he kept putting objects in his mouth, and the nursing staff noticed that he made inappropriate sexual comments. Based on these behavioral changes, what structures of his brain were damaged by his illness?
A. Frontal lobes
B. Temporal lobes
C. Occipital lobes
D. Corpus callosum
E. Substantia nigra

21. A 45-year-old woman brings her elderly mother to see you because she is concerned about her behavior. She states that her mother has been forgetful, gets lost easily, and requires help with self-care. Recently, she has been refusing to let her daughter brush her hair, complaining that it hurts. Additionally, the daughter reports that her mother has been refusing food and has lost weight. On exam, you notice that the patient has a swollen, nonpulsatile right temporal artery that is tender to palpation. You admit the patient to the hospital. What would you expect to see on biopsy of this artery?
    A. Granulomatous changes
    B. Deposits of β-amyloid
    C. Atherosclerotic plaques
    D. Normal arterial walls
    E. Aneurysm of temporal artery

22. A 17-year-old gymnast hits the back of his neck on a bar during practice. A CT scan shows a bony fragment protruding into the lateral portion of the dorsal columns. Given this lesion, which of the following functions will most likely be affected?
    A. Proprioception of ipsilateral leg
    B. Sweating of ipsilateral face
    C. Motor control of ipsilateral leg
    D. Vibratory sense of ipsilateral arm
    E. Vibratory sense of contralateral arm

23. A 2-month-old girl was taken to the pediatrician because her mother was concerned that her head seemed too big. On exam, the baby had a large head, widened cranial sutures, a large anterior fontanelle, and distended scalp veins. CT scan showed markedly dilated ventricles. Which of the following is the most likely cause?
    A. Arnold-Chiari malformation
    B. Defective cerebral aqueduct
    C. Spina bifida occulta
    D. Trisomy 21
    E. Anencephaly

24. You are on-call during your medicine rotation and go with your resident to see a patient in the ED. He is a 52-year-old homeless man with a known history of alcoholism. He is confused and agitated, and seems to be hallucinating. Upon exam, you find that he is sweaty, tachycardic, and hypertensive. Your resident tells you to write the medication order for this patient. What is the mechanism of action for the drug you prescribe?
    A. Inhibit sodium channel opening
    B. Inhibit the sodium-potassium ATPase
    C. Increase the duration of GABA-binding chloride channel opening
    D. Increase the frequency of GABA-binding chloride channel opening
    E. Activate opioid receptors

25. You see a young woman in clinic who complains that she is constantly thirsty, and wakes up several times a night to urinate. She has no other urinary symptoms, and has had no change in her appetite. You order lab tests and find that her blood glucose is normal, but her urine osmolality is low. An abnormality in what neurological structure could account for her symptoms?
    A. Putamen
    B. Substantia nigra
    C. Hypothalamus
    D. Pons
    E. Thalamus

1. D

2. C

3. C

4. B

5. B

6. C

7. A

8. C

9. D

10. F

11. C

12. D

13. C

14. C

15. D

16. A

17. B

18. B

19. B

20. B

21. A

22. D

23. B

24. D

25. C

1. Answer: D

This is a classic presentation for an epidural hematoma caused by a blow to the temple that damages the middle meningeal artery. Arterial bleeding results in a rapid accumulation of blood in the epidural space. In contrast, venous bleeding from a sinus or vein would be slow, and symptoms would develop over a longer period. The great vein of Galen (C) is usually not affected by trauma, although it can occasionally undergo thrombosis. Similarly, thrombosis in the cavernous sinus (B) can occur as a result of infections. Hemorrhage from arteries at the base of the brain such as the inferior cerebellar artery (E) produce subarachnoid hemorrhages and are not often linked to trauma. Disruption of blood flow in branches of the external carotid artery (F) typically does not present significant clinical problems, although a lack of flow in the ophthalmic branch may lead to blindness.

2. Answer: C

Plaques and neurofibrillary tangles are typical for Alzheimer's disease, the most common form of senile dementia. The primary regions shown to be affected by Alzheimer's disease include the basal nucleus of Meynert (which contains cholinergic neurons that project widely to the forebrain and the cerebral cortex), the hippocampal formation, and the cerebral cortex. Choice (B) suggests Huntington's disease, in which a significant reduction of acetylcholine (ACh) and GABA is found in the basal ganglia. Loss of pigmentation in the substantia nigra (D) is a hallmark of Parkinson's disease. Amyotrophic lateral sclerosis is characterized by progressive motor weakness as a result of shrinkage and loss of cell bodies in the anterior horn (A). Nonspecific Wallerian degeneration (E) is seen most often in cases of injury.

3. Answer: C

The vagus nerve supplies motor fibers to the palate. With a unilateral lesion to the nerve, the corresponding side of the palate will fail to rise (left, in this patient) and the uvula will be pulled toward the normal side (right). Since the right side of the palate is higher than the left, it may be assumed that the right side is elevated normally. Therefore, there cannot be any damage to the right vagus (D), which innervates the muscles of the right half of the palate. The glossopharyngeal nerve (A and B) does not send motor fibers to the palate. Even though the spinal accessory nerve (E and F) has some motor contribution to striated muscles of soft palate, pharynx and larynx (as a part of vagus), its major affected muscle groups are the sternocleidomastoid and trapezius.

4. Answer: B

About 1% of the population has a berry aneurysm. Rupture of these berry aneurysms (which can occur suddenly) often involve the circle of Willis, with resultant bleeding into the subarachnoid space. The blood may cause irritation and spasm of adjacent arteries (vasospasm) with worsening of symptoms from cerebral ischemia. The LP did not reveal presence of any WBCs, and the patient was afebrile, making an acute purulent process (E) unlikely. PML (C) is a progressive illness in immunocompromised patients caused by the J-C papovavirus and produces neurologic decline over a longer period of time. Creutzfeldt-Jakob disease (A) is caused by an abnormal prion protein—presence of CSF protein 14-3-3 is the gold standard for clinically diagnosing the disease. Huntington's disease (D) is characterized by onset of choreoathetosis and dementia beginning at the latest by the fifth decade of life. A reduction in dopamine metabolites are sometimes found in the CSF of these patients.

5. Answer: B

A TIA is caused by an interruption of blood flow to brain cells that results in decreases in brain function/neurological deficit, with complete resolution of symptoms in under 24 hours. Symptoms vary with the area of the brain affected and may include changes in vision, speech or comprehension, vertigo, decreased movement or sensation in a part of the body, or changes in the level of consciousness. If the blood flow is decreased for a sufficient period, brain cells in the area die (infarct), causing permanent damage. Loss of blood circulation to the brain can be caused by narrowing of a blood vessel (D), blood clotting within an artery of the brain (A), blood clot traveling to the brain from somewhere else in the body [heart (E) and cholesterol emboli from plaques (C)], and inflammation of or injury to blood vessels.

6. Answer: C

This patient has tertiary syphilis (neurosyphilis) with signs of "tabes dorsalis," a parenchymatous neurosyphilis in which there is slowly progressive degeneration of the posterior columns and roots and ganglia of the spinal cord. The condition usually occurs 15–20 years after initial syphilitic infection. Other neurological deficits can include stabbing, lightning pains, urinary incontinence, ataxia, impaired position and vibratory sense, optic atrophy, hypotonia, hyporeflexia, and trophic joint degeneration (Charcot's joints). *Treponema pallidum* infection leads to endarteritis in the brain and aorta, and sometimes also leads to chronic meningitis. Neurosyphilis may lead to neuronal loss in the brain, but not anterior horn cells (A). Anterior horn cell loss is a feature of ALS and of poliomyelitis. Plaques of demyelination in white matter (B) are characteristic for multiple sclerosis. Hemorrhagic encephalitis (D) is more typically seen with herpes simplex virus infections. Spondylotic myelopathy (often cervical; E) is the most common cause of spinal cord dysfunction in the elderly. The aging process results in degenerative changes in the cervical spine that can cause compression of the cord.

7. Answer: A

Huntington's disease is inherited in an autosomal dominant pattern. The gene has been identified on Chromosome 4, and encodes a protein called huntingtin. HD is a basal ganglia disease; the portions most severely affected are the caudate nucleus and putamen—the most significant neuropathologic change is a preferential loss of medium spiny neurons in the neostriatum. It can be diagnosed on MRI by caudate atrophy with appropriate history and by genetic testing (to detect expanding trinucleotide repeats). The locus ceruleus (D) is located in the brainstem and is not selectively affected by neurodegenerative diseases. The cerebellum (B) and corticospinal tract (E) are not usually associated with specific neurodegenerative disorders. The temporal lobe may demonstrate atrophy with Alzheimer's disease, while marked "knife-like" atrophy of frontal and temporal lobes (C) is characteristic for Pick's disease.

8. Answer: C
Wernicke's disease can lead to hemorrhages and/or loss of periaqueductal gray matter. The Wernicke-Korsakoff syndrome is seen most commonly with chronic alcoholism. Pathophysiologic mechanisms are thought to be secondary to thiamine deficiency. The patient's hepatocellular carcinoma was presumably a long-term complication of micronodular cirrhosis from alcoholism. The anatomic pathology of Alzheimer's disease (D) includes cerebrocortical atrophy (predominantly at the expense of association regions), and neurofibrillary tangles and senile plaques at the microscopic level. The co-occurrence of neurofibrillary tangles and senile plaques was described by Alzheimer in his original description of the disorder and now is accepted universally as a hallmark of the disease. However, while these lesions are characteristic of Alzheimer's disease, they are not pathognomonic of the condition. Characteristic lesions of diffuse cortical Lewy body disease (B) is the Lewy body, an eosinophilic (hematoxylin and eosin staining) round inclusion found in the cytoplasm of substantia nigra cells and in the nucleus basalis of Meynert, locus ceruleus, dorsal raphe, and the dorsal motor nucleus of cranial nerve X. Huntington's disease (E) produces atrophy of the caudate nucleus. Chronic subdural hematoma (A) is unlikely to cause insults to specific anatomical regions.

9. Answer: D
The patient's symptoms and the time course are consistent with Guillain-Barré syndrome—an acute, ascending, and progressive neuropathy characterized by weakness, paresthesias, and hyporeflexia. In severe cases, muscle weakness may lead to respiratory failure, requiring urgent intubation and admission to the intensive care unit. Severe labile autonomic dysfunction may also occur. Maximal weakness typically occurs 2 weeks after the initial onset of symptoms but may evolve rapidly and abruptly. In ALS (E), patients often present with weakness and atrophy of the intrinsic hand muscles, hyperreflexia with extensor plantar responses, and clonus. Thigh fasciculations are common. Sensory involvement, if any, is minimal. Myasthenia gravis (A) is a chronic autoimmune neuromuscular disease characterized by varying degrees of weakness of the skeletal muscles of the body. The hallmark is muscle weakness that increases during periods of activity and improves after periods of rest. There is no mention of symptoms to suggest diabetic neuropathy (B) or polyradiculopathy, a rapidly progressive, ascending course often seen in advanced HIV disease and CMV infection (C).

10. Answer: F
Polymyositis is an idiopathic inflammatory myopathy with symmetric proximal muscle weakness, elevated skeletal muscle enzyme levels, and characteristic electromyography and muscle biopsy findings. Dysphagia secondary to oropharyngeal and esophageal involvement occurs in about a third of patients and is a poor prognostic sign; ocular muscles are almost never involved. Clinically similar to polymyositis, dermatomyositis (C) is an idiopathic inflammatory myopathy associated with characteristic dermatologic manifestations. Patients with hyperthyroidism (D) present with fatigue, palpitations, heat intolerance, sweating, nervousness, or increased bowel movements. Lambert-Eaton syndrome (E) is a rare condition in which weakness results from an abnormality of ACh release at the neuromuscular junction. Weakness is the major symptom, with proximal muscles more affected than distal muscles (especially in the lower limbs)—however, usually mild compared to patients' reports. Lupus myopathy (A) is uncommon, and the patient does not present with findings suggestive of SLE (arthralgia, fevers, arthritis, photosensitivity, rashes). Toxoplasmosis (B) occurs in immunocompromised patients, particularly those with AIDS, and most often involves the CNS to produce headaches, focal neurological deficits, and seizures.

11. Answer: C
The constellation of findings are characteristic for a schwannoma, referred to as an acoustic neuroma when cranial nerve VIII is involved. These are benign neoplasms, typically sporadic (and thus not B), and surgical removal is curative. A solitary mass is unlikely to be part of neurofibromatosis (A), although presence of unilateral vestibular neuroma should mandate inclusion of neurofibromatosis type 2 in one's differential diagnosis. The AIDS-related neoplasm (D) seen in the CNS is a high-grade non-Hodgkin's lymphoma. Neoplasms usually do not have remitting courses, but are progressive—remissions and exacerbations (E) are typically seen in multiple sclerosis. The demyelinated plaques are sometimes big enough to mimic a neoplasm.

12. Answer: D
This patient most likely has a *Toxoplasma* infection—an opportunistic infection that occurs commonly in immunocompromised patients, particularly those with AIDS, and most often involves the CNS to produce abscesses that are ring-enhancing on CT or MRI. Toxoplasmosis associated

with HIV infection is typically caused by reactivation of a chronic infection and manifests primarily as toxoplasmic encephalitis. Pyrimethamine (a dihydrofolate reductase inhibitor) is considered the cornerstone in the treatment of toxoplasmosis, and combination treatment with pyrimethamine plus clindamycin has been shown to be effective during the acute phase of therapy. A long course of broad-spectrum antibiotics (A) would be more appropriate for patients with suspected bacterial meningitis or sepsis. A solitary lesion on brain imaging in an HIV patient is usually indicative of a primary CNS lymphoma, in which case cranial radiation and high-dose chemotherapy (C), as well as intensive anti-HIV treatment (B), are the usual therapeutic approaches.

13. Answer: C

Electrolyte disturbances frequently cause encephalopathy. In this case, severe hyponatremia is diagnosed in a patient presenting with delirium. Unfortunately, too rapid a correction of the hyponatremia by aggressive fluid replacement resulted in central pontine myelinolysis, a noninflammatory demyelination within the central basis pontis. The mechanism is thought to be secondary to cellular edema, caused by fluctuating osmotic forces, and subsequent compression of fiber tracts and induction of demyelination—a process called osmotic myelinolysis. Other conditions that predispose patients to central pontine myelinolysis include alcoholism, malnutrition, and liver disease. Watershed infarctions (A) are likely to be the result of severe perfusion failure and not electrolyte abnormalities. Plaques of demyelination (B) are hallmark findings in patients with multiple sclerosis. Spongiform encephalopathy (E) is a feature of Creutzfeldt-Jakob disease, a rapidly progressive dementia caused by abnormal prion protein. Intraparenchymal hemorrhage (D) is usually caused by trauma (brain contusions) or abnormalities of cerebral blood vessels, such as aneurysms or arteriovenous malformations. Subarachnoid hemorrhage (F) is more likely to be a consequence of trauma or ruptured berry aneurysm.

14. Answer: C

This patient has typical symptoms of Duchenne's muscular dystrophy (male, 5 years of age, tip-toe walking, inability to run, Gower's sign). Duchenne's muscular dystrophy is caused by absent or reduced levels of the dystrophin protein, normally encoded by a gene on the short arm of the X chromosome. Actin, myosin, and troponin participate in muscle contraction. Myosin (B) forms the thick filaments in myofibrils, the components of a muscle fiber. Actin (A) forms the thin filaments in myofibrils. During muscle contraction, actin and myosin bind to one another in a process partially regulated by the protein troponin (E). Kinesin (D) is a cytoplasmic protein responsible for intracellular trafficking of vesicles/particles.

15. Answer: D

Because motor output and sensory input are largely controlled by contralateral hemispheres, right-sided weakness and sensory loss already localizes the lesion to the left side of the brain, ruling out (A) and (C). The patient's deficits mostly involve her leg, which is represented medially in the homunculus, in the territory of the anterior cerebral artery (parasagittal cerebral cortex). An occlusion of the middle cerebral artery (A and B) would be more likely to involve language, and motor/sensory to face, hand, and arm. An occlusion of the basilar artery (E) would most likely cause brainstem dysfunction; branches of the basilar artery supply the entire brainstem and cerebellum, the posterior limb of the internal capsule, medial thalamus, and occipital and medial temporal lobes.

16. Answer: A

These signs/symptoms are consistent with multiple sclerosis—she is a woman between 20 and 50, white, complaining of characteristic double vision, with scattered lesions throughout the CNS. In addition to its association with multiple sclerosis, HLA DR2 (A) is also associated with SLE. DR3 (B) is associated with SLE, diabetes mellitus, and Sjögren's syndrome. DR4 (C) is associated with diabetes mellitus. B27 (D) is associated with ankylosing spondylitis and Reiter's syndrome. Lastly, A3 (E) is associated with hemochromatosis.

17. Answer: B

Small cell carcinoma of the lung is associated with Lambert-Eaton syndrome, a condition in which antitumor antibodies cross-react with voltage-gated calcium channels involved in ACh release, resulting in muscle weakness. In contrast to myasthenia gravis (E), the weakness caused by Lambert-Eaton improves if contraction is steadily maintained (allowing ACh to build up). Weakness is prominent in proximal limb muscles, and patients often have difficulty talking, chewing, and swallowing. Lambert-Eaton syndrome can also occur with autoimmune disorders. Although multiple sclerosis (A) can present with muscle weakness, this patient lacks the typical characteristics associated with the illness (he is male and older than the typical age of onset). A brain tumor (C) affecting the motor cortex might cause weakness, but would be unlikely to explain the inconsistent nature of his weakness (it improves with muscle use) and would likely present with other symptoms as well (headache, seizures). Muscle weakness in the setting of a long smoking history does not support the diagnosis of renal failure (D).

18. Answer: B
This patient has classic symptoms of excess parasympathetic activity. Remember DUMBELSS: Diarrhea, Urination, Miosis, Bronchospasm, Excitation, Lacrimation, Sweating, Salivation. Since organophosphate pesticides act as cholinomimetics, toxic exposure would explain these symptoms. Food poisoning (A) and asthma exacerbation (D) would not be associated with autonomic dysfunction. In amphetamine overdose (C), you may see fever, convulsions, decreased urine output, and nausea/vomiting. Although some poisonous mushrooms (E) may stimulate the parasympathetic nervous system, the patient's employment is the clue suggesting pesticides are the culprit.

19. Answer: B
Several clues in this vignette point to Lyme disease (clues: Connecticut, "bull's eye" rash, flu-like symptoms). Acquired by tick bite, infection with the spirochete *Borrelia burgdorferi* may be followed by neurologic symptoms up to 10 weeks later. Neurologic involvement is typically meningitis/meningoencephalitis, and disorders of cranial nerves and peripheral nerves. Cardiac abnormalities may also occur. Although other cranial nerves may be affected, Lyme disease is characteristically associated with Bell's palsy (resulting in paralysis of facial muscles secondary to dysfunction of facial nerve). See Chapter 6, Cranial Nerves, for review of the other cranial nerves listed (A, C, D, and E).

20. Answer: B
Fever, headache, and seizure suggest some sort of CNS infection (meningitis, meningoencephalitis). Lymphocytosis and elevated protein in CSF is consistent with viral etiology, and should cause suspicion for herpes encephalitis, which has a predilection for the temporal lobes. Hyperorality and hypersexuality (along with visual agnosia) are characteristic of Klüver-Bucy syndrome, a rare disorder resulting from ablation of bilateral temporal lobes, making damage to this region of the brain most consistent with the history. Frontal lobe (A) damage can also cause disinhibition, but given the likelihood of herpes encephalitis, and the presence of hyperorality, temporal lobe damage is more likely. Damage to occipital lobes, corpus callosum, or substantia nigra (C, D, E) should not result in behavioral change.

21. Answer: A
This woman's symptoms are consistent with temporal arteritis, a systemic vasculitis of unknown etiology. It is characterized by a granulomatous inflammatory process, mostly involving the internal elastic lamina of arterial walls. (Note: Intradural arteries have no elastic lamina, so cerebral circulation not usually involved.) Biopsy of the temporal artery also shows mononuclear and giant cell infiltration. Inflammation leads to stenosis, and ultimately occlusion of arterial segment. Temporal arteritis must be diagnosed and treated early, since about 60% of cases will progress to blindness if untreated, secondary to ischemic optic neuritis. Symptoms include headache (and sensitivity to anything touching the head, like a comb or brush), temporal artery tenderness, lack of pulse in the affected artery, and constitutional symptoms (malaise, anorexia). Erythrocyte sedimentation rate is elevated. Deposits of β-amyloid (B) are seen extracellulary on brain biopsy in Alzheimer's disease. Atherosclerotic plaque (C) may cause occlusion, but shouldn't cause inflammatory and constitutional symptoms. Given the findings of a swollen, nonpulsatile artery on exam, one would not expect to see normal arterial walls (D) on biopsy. Aneurysm of the temporal artery (E) does not explain inflammatory symptoms, constitutional symptoms, or pain.

22. Answer: D
To answer this question, first recall what information is carried by the dorsal columns, how are they organized, and where the information crosses. The dorsal columns carry discriminative touch, vibratory sense, and proprioception. They are divided into the fasciculus gracilis (information from legs) and fasciculus cuneatus (information from arms). Remember that fibers carrying information from the upper body (arms) are lateral to fibers carrying information from the lower body (legs). Impulses do not cross until after they have synapsed in the medulla; therefore, a lesion in the dorsal columns themselves will result in an ipsilateral deficit. That rules out (E). (B) and (C) are eliminated, because the dorsal columns do not carry autonomic or motor function. Because the lesion is in the lateral portion of the dorsal columns, the fasciculus cuneatus is most likely to be affected, resulting in a deficit in the arm, as opposed to the leg (A).

23. Answer: B
Markedly dilated ventricles suggests hydrocephalus—excess CSF in the ventricular system. This excess fluid increases intracranial pressure, resulting in findings such as distended scalp veins, widened sutures, and enlarged head. Hydrocephalus can be communicating or

noncommunicating. In communicating hydrocephalus, the CSF is able to flow freely between all the ventricles and into the subarachnoid space. However, there may be defective absorption of CSF, overproduction of CSF, or venous drainage insufficiency. In noncommunicating hydrocephalus, flow is obstructed within the ventricular system. A common cause is "aqueductal stenosis," in which the cerebral aqueduct is narrowed and blocks the flow of CSF. The Arnold-Chiari malformation (A) is a congenital abnormality in which the medulla, fourth ventricle, and cerebellum are displaced downwardly into the cervical spinal canal, possibly due to a relatively small posterior fossa. While Arnold-Chiari malformation can cause hydrocephalus, aqueductal stenosis is a more common cause. Spina bifida occulta (C) is the most mild form of the neural tube defects, in which the neural tube fails to completely close during development. Trisomy 21 (D) results in Down's syndrome. Anencephaly (E) is the complete absence of the brain.

24. Answer: D
Given this patient's known history of alcoholism, alcohol withdrawal or delirium tremens is the most likely explanation for his symptoms. Delirium tremens can develop 2–3 days after cessation of alcohol ingestion. Withdrawal of alcohol results in a functional decrease in the inhibitory neurotransmitter GABA, allowing for an unopposed increase in sympathetic activity. The treatment of choice includes benzodiazepines, which have direct effects on GABA-binding chloride channels, resulting in increasing the frequency of opening. Barbiturates increase the duration of channel opening (C). Because the actions of GABA-binding chloride channels are inhibitory, one would not want to reduce their effects by shortening the duration of their opening (A) or reducing the frequency of their opening (B) when the patient is already in a relatively hyperactivated state.

25. Answer: C
Polydipsia and polyuria in the setting of normal blood glucose support the diagnosis of diabetes insipidus, a condition in which the hypothalamus fails to produce adequate antidiuretic hormone (which is stored and released by the pituitary gland), or the kidneys fail to respond to that hormone, resulting in the output of dilute urine. The putamen (A) is part of the basal ganglia; with the caudate nucleus, it forms the striatum. The substantia nigra (B), located in the midbrain, is closely associated with the basal ganglia. These all function in motor control. The pons (D) is located in the brainstem between the midbrain and the medulla. The thalamus (E) receives and processes sensory and motor information, and relays this information to the appropriate regions of the cerebral cortex.

Index

Page numbers in *italics* denote figures; those followed by a *t* denote tables.

Abducens nerve (CN VI), *18, 19,* 25, 64
Abscess, brain, 66, 79, *83*
Accessory nerve (CN XI), *18,* 26
Acetylcholine, 5, 6t, 38, 39, 41t
Acoustic neuroma, 26, 67, 92
Acyclovir, 46, 66
Adenoma, pituitary, 23, 67, *83*
Adrenal glands, *38, 40,* 41t
Adrenergic receptors, *38,* 42
Afferent nerves, 27t, 38, 39, 56
AIDS dementia complex, 74 (*See also* HIV disease)
AIDS-associated myopathies, 72
Akinesia, 54
Alar plate, *9*
Albuterol, 38
Alcohol abuse (*See also* Drug abuse)
    cerebellar dysfunction from, 52, 72–73
    coma from, 20
    fetal alcohol syndrome and, 7
    meningitis and, 65
    peripheral neuropathy from, 47
    pontine myelinolysis from, 93
    seizures from, 59
    subdural hematoma from, 69
    Wernicke's encephalopathy from, 57, 92
    withdrawal from, 60t, 95
Alpha-fetoprotein, 9
ALS (*See* Amyotrophic lateral sclerosis)
Alzheimer's disease, 60t, 73, 90–92
    (*See also* Dementia)
Amaurosis fugax, 74, 75t
Amikacin, 72
Aminoglycosides, 46, 72
Amnesia, 57, 86, 89
Amniocentesis, 9
Amphetamines, 94
Amygdala, *53,* 57
Amyloid precursor protein, 73
Amyotrophic lateral sclerosis (ALS), 91, 92
Anemia, pernicious, 34
Anencephaly, 9t
Anesthesia, saddle, 29
Anesthetic
    general, 59, 72
    local, 4
Aneurysm, rupture of, 69, 91
Angiography, *78–81*
Angioma, 79
Anorexia, 56
Anosmia, 23
Anterior inferior cerebellar artery (AICA), 12, *21,* 21t
Anticholinergics, 41
Anticonvulsants, 52, 59–61
Antidepressants, 5, 59
Antidiuretic hormone (ADH), 42, 56, 95

Antimuscarinics, 41
Antinicotinics, 41
Aphasia, 13, 75
Apnea, sleep, 62
Apoplexy, pituitary, 67
Apraxia, 50
Arachnoid granulations, 64
Arachnoid mater, 9, 63
Argyll-Robertson pupil, 66
Arnold-Chiari malformation, 9f, 47, 64, 95
Arteritis, temporal, 94
Astrocytes, 1, 68
Ataxia, 72, 75t, 91
    anticonvulsants and, 60
    Friedreich's, 52, 73
    Kearns-Sayre-Daroff syndrome and, 71
    Wernicke's encephalopathy and, 57
Ataxia-telangiectasia, 73
Atenolol, 42
Atherosclerosis, 94
    risks for, 11
    stroke from, 12, 74, 75
Athetosis, 54
Atrial septal defect, 7
Atropine toxicity, 41
Auditory cortex, 13, 46
Auerbach's plexus, 42
Autonomic nervous system (ANS), 37–42, *40,* 41t, 56
Axodendritic synapse, 5
Axons, 1, 2f (*See also* Neurons)

Babinski's sign, 32–34
Balance disorders, 46, 72–73, 75t
Barbiturates, 6
Basal ganglia, 53–54, 95
Basal plate, *9*
Basilar artery, *11, 12, 21,* 21t
Becker's dystrophy, 71
Belladonna, 41
Bell's palsy, 26, 94
Benign febrile convulsions of childhood, 59–60, 60t
Benign prostatic hypertrophy, 42
Benzodiazepines, 6, 95
Bladder innervation, 29, *40*
Blindness
    psychic, 57
    after stroke, 21, 74, 75t
    temporal arteritis and, 94
    visual pathway lesions and, *24*
Blood-brain barrier (BBB), 1, 11, 63
Botulism, 5
Bovine spongiform encephalopathy, 74, 93
Brachial plexus, 35
Bradykinesia, 54
Bradykinins, 43

Brain
    abscess in, 66, 79, *83*
    anatomy of, *11–15,* 11–16, *17*
    embryology of, *8*
    gray matter of, 12, *63,* 78
    herniation of, 23, 64, 67
    imaging of, *77–84*
    limbic system of, *55*
    tumor in, 60t, 67–69, *68,* 73, 77, *82*
    vasculature of, *11–12, 21,* 21t, 79
    ventricles of, 14, *15,* 64, *65, 68,* 78
    white matter of, 12, 14, 78
Brainstem
    anatomy of, *17–21*
    motor areas of, 50, *51, 54*
    sleep apnea and, 62
Breast cancer, 82
Broca's area, *13,* 75
Brodmann's areas, 49
Brown-Séquard's syndrome, *34*

Calcifications, cerebral, 10t, 77
Calcium channels, 5, 61
Carotid arteries, *11, 12, 21,* 75t, 90
    angiography of, *78–81*
    cavernous sinuses and, *25*
Carpal tunnel syndrome, 35
Cataplexy, 62
Cataracts, congenital, 10t
Cauda equina, 29
Caudate nucleus, *14,* 53, *54,* 91, 95
Ceftriaxone, 66
Central core disease, 71
Cerebellopontine angle, 26, 87
Cerebellum, *15, 17,* 51–52
    anticonvulsants and, 60
    degeneration of, 72–73
    embryology of, *8*
    metastases in, *82*
    spinal tracts and, 46, *51, 52, 54*
    vasculature of, *11, 12, 21,* 21t
Cerebral arteries, *11, 12, 21,* 21t
    motor cortex and, 49
    occlusion of, 74, 75t, 93
Cerebrospinal fluid (CSF), 1, 94, 95
    evaluation of, 66t
    imaging of, *79*
    increased ICP and, *68*
    intracranial hemorrhage and, 69
    lumbar puncture and, 63–64, *64,* 85
Cerebrovascular accidents (*See* Strokes)
Cerebrum (*See* Brain)
Charcot's joints, 91
Chicken pox virus, 25, 46
Child abuse, 69
Cholinergic neuron, *39*
Cholinesterase inhibitors, 73

Cholinomimetics, 41
Chorda tympani, 25
Chorea, 54
Choroid plexus, 64, 65, 77
Ciliary ganglion, *24*
Cinchonism, 26, 72
Cingulate gyrus, 12, *55*, 57
Ciprofloxacin, 66
Circadian rhythms, 56
Circle of Willis, *11, 12, 21,* 69
Cirrhosis, 65
Clark's column, 46
Claw-hand deformity, 35
Clindamycin, 93
Clonus, 33t, 59
Cluster headache, 61
CN (*See* Cranial nerves)
Coagulopathy, 74
Cocaine, 4, 5 (*See also* Drug abuse)
Coccygeal root, *30*
Cochlear nerve (*See* Vestibulocochlear nerve)
Colloid cyst, 69
Colorectal cancer, *82*
Coma
  causes of, 20
  encephalitis and, 66
  stroke and, 75t
  Wernicke's encephalopathy and, 57
Computed tomography (CT), 77, *78–82*
Conus medullaris, 29
Convulsions (*See* Seizures)
Copper metabolism, 54
Corpus callosum, 12, *14*
Corticobulbar tract, 49, *54*
Corticospinal tract, *18, 19,* 31, *32,* 49–50, *51, 54*
Coxsackievirus, 66
Cranial nerves (CN), *11,* 17–18, *18–20,* 23–27
  functions of, 27t
  Lyme disease and, 66
  mnemonics for, 23, 27
  tumors of, 26, 67, 92
Cranial nerve I (*See* Olfactory nerve)
Cranial nerve II (*See* Optic nerve)
Cranial nerve III (*See* Oculomotor nerve)
Cranial nerve IV (*See* Trochlear nerve)
Cranial nerve V (*See* Trigeminal nerve)
Cranial nerve VI (*See* Abducens nerve)
Cranial nerve VII (*See* Facial nerve)
Cranial nerve VIII (*See* Vestibulocochlear nerve)
Cranial nerve IX (*See* Glossopharyngeal nerve)
Cranial nerve X (*See* Vagus nerve)
Cranial nerve XI (*See* Accessory nerve)
Cranial nerve XII (*See* Hypoglossal nerve)
Craniopharyngioma, 69
Creutzfeldt-Jakob disease, 74, 91, 93
"Crocodile tears," 26
Cryptococcosis, 66
CSF (*See* Cerebrospinal fluid)
Cyst, colloid, 69
Cysticercosis, 66
Cytomegalovirus, 10t

Dantrolene, 72
Deafness (*See* Hearing loss)
Delirium, 93
Delirium tremens, 95
Dementia, 60t, 73–74, 90–93
  practice questions on, 85, 86
  subdural hematoma and, *82*
Demyelination, 1, 63, 74 (*See also* Multiple sclerosis)
  cerebellar, 52
  peripheral neuropathy with, 47
  pontine, 93
  spinal, 34
Dermatomes, *25, 31*
Dermatomyositis, 72
Diabetes insipidus, 56, 95
Diabetes mellitus, 11, 47, 65, 74
Diazepam, 59
Diencephalon, *8,* 14–16, 16t, *17*
Diplopia, 23, 25, 50, 93
Donepezil, 73
Dopa decarboxylase, 5
Dopamine, 5, 42
  basal ganglia and, 53, 54
  memory and, 58
  properties of, 6t
Dorsal columns, *32, 34, 45,* 94
Dorsal root ganglion, 1, *9, 37,* 38, 43
Double vision, 23, 25, 50, 93
Down's syndrome, 9, 73
Drug abuse, 60t, 66, 94 (*See also* Alcohol abuse)
  cocaine and, 4, 5
  dementia and, 73
  opiates and, 20
Duchenne's dystrophy, 71, 93
Dura mater, 63
Dysarthria
  cerebellar lesion and, 52, 73
  nucleus ambiguous and, 20
Dysphagia, 20, 86–87
  myasthenia gravis and, 6
  stroke and, 75t

Echovirus, 66
Eclampsia, 60t
Ectoderm, 7, 9
Edema, cerebral, 77, 78, *81*
Edinger-Westphal nucleus, *18, 24,* 39
Edrophonium, 6
Edwards' syndrome, 9
Efferent nerves, 27t, *37,* 38, 56
Ehlers-Danlos syndrome, 69
Electrical potential, 2–3, *4*
Electrolyte disturbances, 93
Embryology, 7–9, 9t, 10t
Encephalitis, 66, 93
  coma from, 20
  CSF in, 66t
  herpes, 10t, 91, 94
  Lyme disease and, 94
  seizures from, 60t
  sleep apnea and, 62
Encephalopathy
  hepatic, 60t
  HIV, 60t, 74

spongiform, 74, 93
  Wernicke's, 57, 92
Endocarditis, 66, 75
Endocytosis, 5
Enteric nervous system, 42
Entorhinal cortex, *55, 56,* 57
Ependymoma, 69
Epidural hematoma, 69, 90
Epilepsy, 20, 56, 59–61, 60t (*See also* Seizures)
  brain tumor and, 67
  MERRF syndrome and, 72
  uncinate, 23
Epinephrine, 6t, 42
Epstein-Barr virus (EBV), 66
Equilibrium disorders, 46, 72–73, 75t
Equilibrium potential, 2–3, *3, 4*
Erb's palsy, 35
Ergotamine, 61
Esmolol, 42
Exocytosis, 5

Facial nerve (CN VII), *18, 19,* 25–26
  Bell's palsy and, 26
  Horner's syndrome and, 38
  Lyme disease and, 66, 94
  parasympathetic nervous system and, *39, 40*
Falx cerebri, *67*
Faraday constant, 3
Fasciculations, 33t, 92
Fasciculus cuneatus, *32, 45,* 94
Fasciculus gracilis, *32, 45,* 94
Fatal familial insomnia, 74
Febrile convulsions, 59–60, 60t
Fetal alcohol syndrome, 7
α-Fetoprotein, 9
Fight or flight response, 38
Filum terminale, 29
Floppy baby syndrome, 5
Folate deficiency, 7, 9, 47
Forebrain, *8,* 9, *17*
Friedreich's ataxia, 52, 73
Frontal lobe, *13,* 94

Gag reflex, 26
Gait disturbance, 53, 71, 72, 87
Gamma-aminobutyric acid (GABA), 6, 53, 54, 95
Gap junctions, 5
Gaze center, *19*
Gentamicin, 46, 72
Giant cells, 94
Glial cells, 1
Glioblastoma multiforme, 67
Glioma, 67, *82*
Globus pallidus, *14,* 53
Glossopharyngeal nerve (CN IX), *18, 20,* 26, *39, 40*
Glutamate, 53
Glycine, 6
Gottron's papules, 72
Gowers' sign, 71, 93
Granule cells, 57
Gray communicant rami, *37*
Gray matter, 79

cerebral, 12, *63*, *78*
periaqueductal, 18
spinal, 9, *30*, 31, 39, *78*
Guillain-Barré syndrome, 92

Hallucinations, 62
Halothane, 72
Hand innervation, *31*, *35*, 47
Head trauma
epidural hematoma from, 69, 90
imaging of, 79
meningitis and, 65
seizures from, 60t
Headaches, 61–62, 64, 88, 94
Hearing loss, 46, 72
rubella and, 10t
tinnitus with, 87
vestibulocochlear nerve and, 26
Heart disease, congenital, 7, 10t
Heliotrope rash, 72
Hemangioblastoma, 69
Hemianopsia
from pituitary adenoma, 23, 67
from stroke, 75t
from visual pathway lesion, *24*
Hemiballismus, 54
Hemiparesis, 50, 75t
Hemiplegia, 50, 75t
Heparin, 75
Hepatolenticular degeneration, 54
Herniation, uncal, 23, 64, 67
Herpes simplex, 10t, 46, 66, 91, 94
Herpes zoster, 25, 46
Hexamethonium, 41
Hindbrain, *8*, *17*
Hippel-Lindau syndrome, 69
Hippocampus, *55*, 56, *57*, 58
Hirschsprung's disease, 9
Histamine, 43
HIV disease, 87, 92–93
CD4 receptors and, 1
dementia from, 74
meningitis and, 65, 66
myopathies of, 72
peripheral neuropathy from, 47
seizures from, 60t
Homeostasis, 56
Homunculus, motor, 31, *49*, 93
Horner's syndrome, 38, 47, 75t
Huntington's disease, 54, 91
Hydrocephalus, 64, 73, 94–95
colloid cyst with, 69
imaging of, 77, *81*
Hypercholesterolemia, 11
Hyperkinesia, 54
Hyperlipidemia, 74
Hyperorality, 94
Hyperosmolar states, 60t
Hyperreflexia, 33t
Hyperthermia, 59–60, 60t, 71, 72
Hyperthyroidism, 92
Hypnagogic hallucinations, 62
Hypocalcemia, 60t
Hypoglossal nerve (CN XII), *18*, *20*, 26
Hypokinesia, 54
Hyponatremia, 60t, 93
Hypothalamus, 14, *17*

autonomic nervous system and, 42
diabetes insipidus and, 95
limbic system and, 56, 57
Hypothyroidism, 52, 73

ICP (*See* Intracranial pressure)
Imaging, *68*, *77–84*
Incontinence, 29, 85, 88, 91
Intention tremor, 52
Internal capsule, *14*
Interneuron, *3*
Intracranial hemorrhage, 60t, 64, 69, 74, 75, *82*
Intracranial pressure (ICP), 67, *68*
headache from, 61–62
hydrocephalus and, 94–95
Ion channels, 2–3, *3*
Isoproterenol, 42

Jacksonian march, 59
Jugular foramen, 26
Junctions, neuromuscular, 6t

Kanamycin, 72
Kayser-Fleischer rings, 54
Kearns-Sayre-Daroff syndrome, 71
Ketoacidosis, 11
Kinesin, 93
Klumpke's palsy, 35
Klüver-Bucy syndrome, 57, 94
Korsakoff's syndrome, 24, 92
Kuru, 74

Labetalol, 42
Lacrimation, 26, 41, 94
Lacunar infarct, 12
Lambert-Eaton syndrome, 5, 92, 93
Lateral geniculate nucleus (LGN), 23, *24*
Lentiform nuclei, 53, 54
Leptomeninges, 63
Leukemia, 73
Lewy bodies, 53, 92
Lidocaine, 4
Light reflexes, 23
Limbic system, 14, *55*, 55–58, *57*
Lipohyalinosis, 11
Lissauer's tract, 43, 44
Lithium, 56
Locked-in syndrome, 75t
Lorazepam, 59
Lumbar puncture, 63–64, *64*, 85 (*See also* Cerebrospinal fluid)
Lung cancer, 5, *82*
Lupus, 92, 93
Luschka, foramen of, 64, 65
Lyme disease, 66, 94
Lymphoma, 73, 92, 93

Mad cow disease, 74
Magendie, foramen of, 64, 65
Magnetic resonance imaging (MRI), 78–79, *79*, *84*
ring enhancements on, *83*, 92
Malignant hyperthermia, 71, 72
Mammillary bodies, *18*
alcohol abuse and, 72
discoloration of, 86

limbic system and, 56, *57*
Marfan's syndrome, 69
Mass effect on imaging, *68*, 77, *82*
Mastication, 23
Measles, 66
Medial lemniscus, *18–20*
Medial longitudinal fasciculus (MLF), *19*, 20
Medulla oblongata, *17–20*, 49
nociception and, *44*, *45*
structures of, 20
vasculature of, 21
Medulloblastoma, 69
Meissner's corpuscle, *43*
Meissner's plexus, 42
Melanocytes, 9
MELAS syndrome, 72
Membrane potential, 2–3, *3*, *4*
Memory, 56–58, 73, 86, 89
Ménière's disease, 72
Meninges, 9t, *63*
Meningioma, 67
intracranial, *82*
spinal, *83*
Meningitis, 63–66
causes of, 65t, 91
CSF in, 66t
hydrocephalus from, 64
Lyme disease and, 94
seizures from, 60t
signs of, 64
Meningocele, 9f
Mental retardation, 10t
Merkel's discs, *43*
MERRF syndrome, 72
Mesencephalon, *8*, 9
Mesolimbic dopaminergic pathway, 58
Metabolic disorders, 60t, 73
Metoprolol, 42
Meyer's loop, 23, *24*
Midbrain, 14–16, 16t, *17*, 21t, 95
cranial nerves of, *18*, *19*
embryology of, *8*
structures of, *18*
visual pathway and, *24*
Migraine, 61
Miosis, *24*, 38, *40*, 41t
Mitochondrial myopathies, 71–72
MLF (*See* Medial longitudinal fasciculus)
Monoamine oxidase inhibitors, 5
Mononuclear cells, 94
Monro, foramen of, 14, 64, 65
Motor cortex, 13, *49–50*, 53, 54
Motor homunculus, 31, *49*, 93
Motor neurons, *3*, 9, 29, *30* (*See also* Neurons)
cranial nerves and, 27t
lesions of, 26, 33t
neuromuscular junction of, 6t
Motor pathways, *32*
Multiple sclerosis, 79, *84*
cerebellar dysfunction from, 52
trigeminal neuralgia and, 61
vision loss from, 19, 24
Mumps, 66
Muscarinic receptors, 6t
Muscular dystrophy, 71, 93

Myasthenia gravis, 6, 92
Mydriasis, *40*, 41t
Myelin sheath, 1, *2*, 34 (*See also* Demyelination)
Myelinolysis, osmotic, 93
Myenteric plexus, 42
Myopathies, 71–72

Narcolepsy, 62
Neck
    imaging of, *77*, *78*, *80*, *83*, *84*
    multiple sclerosis of, *84*
    stiffness of, 64
    trauma to, 89
Nemaline myopathy, 71
Neomycin, 26
Neostigmine, 6
Nernst equation, 3
Neural crest cells, 7, 9
Neural plate, 7
Neural signaling, 2–4, *3*, *4*
Neural tube, 7, *8*, 9t
Neuritic plaques, 73
Neuroblasts, 9
Neurofibrillary tangles, 73
Neurofibromatosis, 26, 67, 92
Neuroma, acoustic, 26, 67, 92
Neuromuscular junctions, 6t
Neuromuscular spindles, 43
Neurons, 1, *2* (*See also* Sensory neurons)
    adrenergic sympathetic, *38*
    cholinergic, *39*
    membrane potential of, 2–3, *3*, *4*
    synapses of, *5*, 6t
Neuropathy, peripheral, 35, 47
Neuropore (*See* Neural tube)
Neurosyphilis
    congenital, 10t
    dementia from, 73
    tabes dorsalis from, 34, 66, 91
Neurotransmitters, 1, *5*, 6, 43
    in autonomic nervous system, 38, 39
    properties of, 6t
Nociceptors, 20, 43
Node of Ranvier, 1, *2*
Norepinephrine, 5, 6t, 38, 41t, 42
Nucleus accumbens, 58
Nucleus ambiguous, *20*
Nucleus cuneatus, 20, *45*
Nucleus gracilis, 20, *45*
Nucleus solitarius (*See* Tractus solitarius)
Nystagmus, 26, 52, 73, 75t

Occipital lobe, *13*, 21t
Oculomotor nerve (CN III), *18*, 23, 24, *39*, *40*
Odontoblasts, 9
Olfactory nerve (CN I), *18*, 23, 57
Oligodendrocytes, 1
Oliva, *20*, 52
Ophthalmoplegia, 57
Opiates, 20 (*See also* Drug abuse)
Optic chiasm, *11*, *18*, 23, *24*, *25*
Optic nerve (CN II), 1, *18*, 23, *24*, 94
Organ of Corti, 46
Organophosphate pesticides, 94
Osmoreceptors, 56

Osmotic myelinolysis, 93
Otitis media, 65
Ototoxicity, 46
Oxytocin, 42, 56

Pacinian corpuscles, *43*
Palsy, 35
    abducens nerve, 64
    Bell's, 26, 94
    cranial nerve, 66
    facial nerve, 26
    supranuclear, 53
Pancoast tumor, 38
Papez circuit, 56, *57*
Papilledema, 62, 64, 67, 85
Paralysis
    facial, 26
    flaccid, 5
    sleep, 62
    spastic, 32
    Todd's, 59
Parasympathetic nervous system, 26, 27t, 38–42, *40*, 41t
Parietal lobe, *13*
Parkinson's disease, 6t, 41, 53, 91
Parotid glands, 26
Paroxysmal disorders, 59–62, 60t
Penicillamine, 54
Penicillin G, 66
Peripheral nerves
    anatomy of, 29–34
    cutaneous receptors of, *43*
    disorders of, 34–35, *35*, 47
Periventricular lucency, *81*
Pesticides, 41, 94
Pharyngioma, 69
Phenelzine, 5
Phenobarbital, 59
Phenoxybenzamine, 42
Phentolamine *N*-methyltransferase, 5
Phenylephrine, 38, 42
Phenytoin, 59, 61
Pia mater, 9, 63
Pick's disease, 73–74, 92
Pineal gland, 77
Pituitary, 14, 56, 95
    adenoma of, 23, 67, *83*
    autonomic nervous system and, 42
    cavernous sinuses and, *25*
Pneumonia, 65
Poisoning, 4, 41, 94
Poliomyelitis, 62, 91
Polycythemia, 74
Polymyositis, 72, 92
Pons, *11*, *17*, *19*, 21t
    myelinolysis of, 93
    nociception and, *44*
    tegmentum of, 23
Porphyria, 60t
Posterior inferior cerebellar artery (PICA), *11*, 12, *21*, 75t
Potassium channels, *3*, *4*
Pott's disease, 66
Pralidoxime, 41
Prazosin, 42
Primary motor cortex, 49–50
Primethamine, 93

Primitive neuroectodermal tumor (PNET), 69
Prion disease, 60t, 74
Procaine, 4
Progressive multifocal leukoencephalopathy (PML), 74, 91
Prolactinoma, 67
Pronator drift, 33t, 49
Propanolol, 42, 61
Proprioception, 34, *51*, 94
Prosencephalon, 8, *9*
Prostaglandins, 43
Prostatic hypertrophy, 42
Psammoma bodies, 67
Ptosis, 6, 38
Puffer fish toxin, 4
Pupils, *40*, 41t
    Argyll-Robertson, 66
    cranial nerves and, *24*, *25*
Purkinje cells, 52
Putamen, *14*, 53, *54*, 91, 95
Pyramidal cell, *3*, *57*
Pyramidal tracts, *18*, *20*, 31, *32*, 49

Quadrantanopsia, *24*
Quadriplegia, 75t
Quinine, 26, 72

Radial palsy, 35
Radiation treatment, 62
Radiculopathy syndromes, 34
Ragged red fibers, 71, 72
Ranvier, node of, 1, *2*
Recombinant tissue plasminogen activator (r-tPA), 75
Red nucleus, *18*, 50, *52*
Reflex(es), 20, 33t, 52
    gag, 26
    light, 23
    stretch, *31*, 32, 33t, 43
Resting potential, *3*, *4*
Reticular activating system (RAS), 20, 62
Reticular formation, 20, *44*, 50
Reticulospinal tract, 50, *51*, *54*
Retinal bipolar cells, 1
Retinopathy, 10t
Reversible ischemic neurological deficit (RIND), 74
Rhombencephalon, 8, *9*
Rifampin, 66
Ring enhancements, on MRI, *83*, 92
Rivastigmine, 73
Rod-shaped bodies, 71
Romberg's sign, 34
Rosenthal fibers, 68
Rubella, 10t
Rubrospinal tract, *32*, 50, *51*, *52*, *54*
Ruffini endings, *43*
Ryanodine receptors, 72

Sacral nerve cells, 39
SAH (*See* Subarachnoid hemorrhage)
Salicylates, 72
Salivation, *40*, 41, 93
    Bell's palsy and, 26
    innervation of, *25*
"Saturday night palsy," 35

Schwann cells, 1, *2*, 9
Schwannoma, 26, 67, 92
Sclerosis (*See* Multiple sclerosis)
Seizures, 59–61, 60t (*See also* Epilepsy)
  congenital infections with, 10t
  meningitis with, 66
  types of, 59
Selective serotonin reuptake inhibitors
  (SSRIs), 5
Sensory neurons, *3*, 9, 29, *30*, 44 (*See also*
  Motor neurons)
  cranial nerves and, 27t
  types of, 43
Sensory pathways, *32*, 43–46, 54
Septum pellucidum, *14*
Serotonin, 5, 6t, 20
Sheehan's syndrome, 67
Shingles, 25, 46
Shunt, ventriculoperitoneal, 64
Sickle cell disease, 74
Sinusitis, 65
SLE (*See* Systemic lupus erythematosus)
Sleep disorders, 62, 74
Sleep regulation, 20, 50, 56
Sodium channels, *3*, 4
Spastic paresis, 32
Spinal accessory nerve (*See* Accessory
  nerve)
Spinal cord
  anatomy of, 29–32, *30–32*
  ascending tracts of, 43–46, *44–46*
  autonomic nervous system and, 37–38
  congenital abnormalities of, 9t
  CSF and, 63–64, *65*
  descending tracts of, 50, *51*, 54
  embryology of, 7–9
  gray matter of, 9, *30*, 31, 39, *78*
  lesions of, *34*
  multiple sclerosis of, *84*
  tumor of, *83*
  vasculature of, *11*, 31, *34*
  vertebrae and, *30*
  white matter of, 9, *30*, 31, *78*
Spinocerebellar tract, *46*, *51*, 52
Spinothalamic tracts, *18*, 20, *32*, 43–47,
  44, 45
Spongiform encephalopathy, 74, 93
Status epilepticus, 59 (*See also* Epilepsy)
Streptomycin, 26, 72
Stretch reflexes, *31*, 32, 33t, 43
Striatum, *53*, 95
Strokes, 20, 74–75, 75t
  cerebellum and, 52
  imaging of, 77, 79, *80*
  management of, 75
  meningitis and, 66
  motor cortex and, 50
  risks for, 74
  seizures from, 60t
  sleep apnea and, 62
  subdural hematoma and, 69
  TIAs and, 74, 75, 86, 91
  types of, *12*, 74
Stylopharyngeus muscle, 26
Subacute combined degeneration of spinal
  cord, *34*
Subacute sclerosing panencephalitis, 66

Subarachnoid hemorrhage (SAH), 60t, 63,
  64, 69, 74, *81*, 90
Subarachnoid space, *63*, *65*
Subdural hematoma, 69, *82*
Subiculum, *56*, *57*
Submucosal plexus, 42
Substance abuse (*See* Drug abuse)
Substance P, 43
Substantia nigra, 6t, *18*, *53*, 54, 95
Subthalamic nucleus (STN), *53*, 54
Succinylcholine, 72
Sumatriptan, 61
Supplementary motor cortex (SMC), 49,
  50
Suprachiasmatic nucleus, 56
Sylvian fissure, 12, *13*
Sympathetic nervous system, 37–38, *40*,
  41t
Sympathomimetics, 42
Synapses, *5*, 6t
Syphilis (*See* Neurosyphilis)
Syringomyelia, *34*, 47
Systemic lupus erythematosus (SLE), 92,
  93

Tabes dorsalis, *34*, 66, 91
Tegmentum, 16
Telangiectasia, 73
Telencephalon, 8, *17*
Temporal arteritis, 94
Temporal lobe, *13*, 46
  imaging of, *78*
  Klüver-Bucy syndrome and, 57, 94
  limbic system and, 55
  necrosis of, 66
  seizures of, 59, *60*
  uncal herniation and, 23, 64, 67
  visual pathway lesions in, *24*
Tension headache, 61
Tentorium cerebelli, 67
Tetrodotoxin, 4
Thalamus, 14, *14*, *15*, 16t, *17*, 21t, 95
  basal ganglia and, *53*, 54
  cerebellar deep nuclei and, 52
  dorsal columns and, 32
  lateral geniculate nucleus of, *24*
  limbic system and, 55, 55–56, *57*
  spinal tracts to, 43–46, *44, 45*
Thiamine deficiency, 57, 73, 92
Thoracic outlet syndrome, 35
Thymus disorders, 6
Thyroid disorders, 52, 73, 92
TIAs (*See* Transient ischemic attacks)
Tic douloureux, 61
Timolol, 42
Tinel's sign, 35
Tinnitus, 72, 87
Tissue plasminogen activator (tPA), 75
Tobramycin, 72
Todd's paralysis, 59
Tongue innervation, 26
TORCHeS syndrome, 10t
Tourette's syndrome, 55
Toxoplasmosis, 10t, 66, 92–93
Tractus solitarius, *20*, 26
Transient ischemic attacks (TIAs), 74, 75,
  86, 91 (*See also* Strokes)

Transtentorial herniation, 23, 64, 67
Tremor, intention, 52
Tricyclic antidepressants, 5
Trigeminal nerve (CN V), *18–20*,
  23–25
  dermatomes of, *25*
  headache and, 61
  herpes and, 25, 46
  sensory pathway of, 46
  tumor of, 61
Trisomy 18, 9
Trisomy 21, 9, 73
Trochlear nerve (CN IV), *18*, 23
Tuberculosis, 65, 66t
Tubocurarine, 41
Tyramine, 5
Tyrosine, 5, 6t

Ulnar neuropathy, 35
Uncal herniation, 23, 64, 67
Uremia, 20, 60t
Uvular deviation, 85, 91

Vagus nerve (CN X), *18*, *20*, 26
  lesion of, 85
  parasympathetic nervous system and, 39,
  40, 42
Valproate, 61
Valsalva maneuver, 34
Varicella, 25, 46
Vasculitis, 63, 94
Vasopressin, 42, 56, 95
Ventricles, cerebral, 14, *15*, 64, *65*,
  68, *78*
Ventriculoperitoneal shunt, 64
Vertebrae, *30*, 66 (*See also* Spinal cord)
Vertebral arteries, *11*, *12*, *21*, 31
Vertigo, 46, 72–73, 75t
Vestibular disorders (*See* Equilibrium
  disorders)
Vestibular nuclei, 50, *52*
Vestibulocochlear nerve (CN VIII), *18–20*,
  26
  schwannoma of, 26, 67, 92
  sensory pathway of, 46
Vestibulospinal tract, 50, *51*, *52*, 54
Visual cortex, 12, 21, *24*
Visual pathways, *24* (*See also* Blindness)
Vitamin B$_1$ deficiency, 57, 73, 92
Vitamin B$_{12}$ deficiency, 34, 47, 73

Wallenberg's syndrome, 75t
Warfarin, 75
Wernicke's area, *13*, 75
Wernicke's syndrome, 57, 92
White communicant rami, *37*
White matter, 79
  cerebral, 12, 14, *78*
  spinal, 9, *30*, 31, *78*
Willis, circle of, *11*, *12*, *21*, 69
Wilson's disease, 54
Withdrawal syndromes, 60t, 95 (*See also*
  Alcohol abuse)

X-rays, 77

Zoster ophthalmicus, 46